Pumping Iron II: The Unprecedented Woman

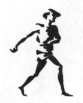

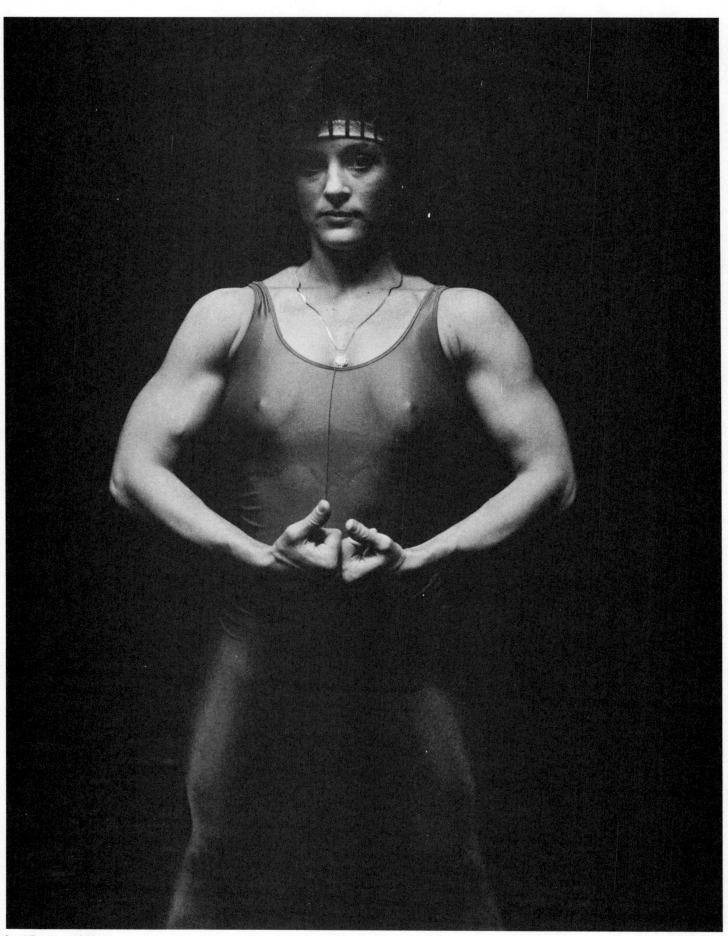

Lori Bowen, 1983

Pumping Iron II:
The Unprecedented Woman

Written by
Charles Gaines

Photographs by
George Butler

Designed by Martin Stephen Moskof

Simon and Schuster   New York

Also by Charles Gaines and George Butler
PUMPING IRON
STAYING HARD
CHARLES ATLAS

Also by Charles Gaines
STAY HUNGRY
DANGLER

Also by George Butler (with David Thorne)
THE NEW SOLDIER

ACKNOWLEDGMENTS

Len Archambault
Jan Bagley
Doris Barrilleaux
Lawrence Chong
Wayne and Karen De Milia
Susan Fry
Eddie Giulianni
Joe Gold
Bernard Heng
Nick Irens
Julie Levine
Cheryl Moch
Andy Olsen
B. S. Ong
Zabo the Renowned
Arnold Schwarzenegger
Franz Stampfl
Stone's Gym
Al Thomas
Tom and Oliver Vaughan
Ben and Joe Weider
David Yaffe,
Ninette Trading Co., Melbourne, Australia

Published by Simon and Schuster,
A Division of Simon & Schuster, Inc.
Simon & Schuster Building, Rockefeller Center,
1230 Avenue of the Americas, New York, New York 10020.

SIMON AND SCHUSTER and colophon
are registered trademarks of Simon & Schuster, Inc.
Design: Martin Moskof Associates, Inc.
Production: Jeanne Palmer

Manufactured in the United States of America

1   3   5   7   9   10   8   6   4   2

Library of Congress Cataloging in Publication Data

Gaines, Charles, date.
Pumping iron II: the unprecedented woman.

1. Bodybuilding for women.   I. Butler, George,
date.   II. Title.
GV546.6.W64G34   1984   646.7′5   83-521
ISBN 0-671-44104-3
0-671-44105-1 Pbk.

To Hansell Gaines Burke,
who knows all about development,
and
Dyanna Taylor
of
Star Hill and Steep Ravine

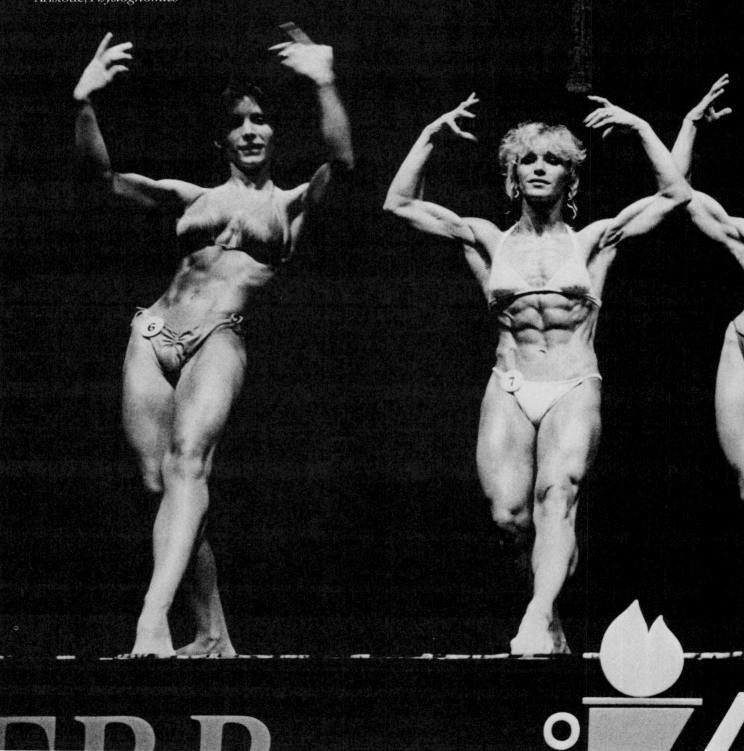

"The author of nature gave man strength of body and intrepidity of mind to enable him to face great hardships, and to woman was given a weak and delicate constitution, accompanied by a natural softness and modest timidity, which fit her for sedentary life."
—Aristotle, *Physiognomics*

"Woman is defective and accidental . . . a male gone awry . . . the result of some weakness in the father's generative power . . ."
—St. Thomas Aquinas

"I will make you acquainted with the proportions of a man; I omit those of a woman, because there is not one of them perfectly proportioned."
—Author (unknown) of a Renaissance treatise on painting

Miss Olympia Competition, 1980

"... but separately, as helpmate, the woman herself alone is not the image of God; whereas the man alone is the image of God as fully and completely as when the woman is joined with him."
—St. Augustine

"Women have served all these centuries as looking glasses possessing the magic and delicious power of reflecting the figure of man at twice its natural size."
—Virginia Woolf, *A Room of One's Own*

"The Nakedness of Woman is the work of God."
—William Blake

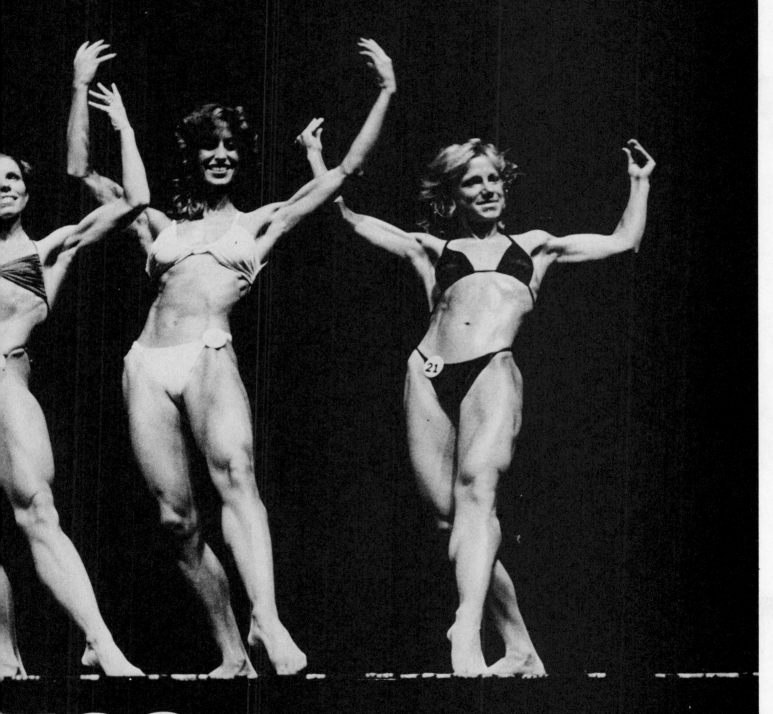

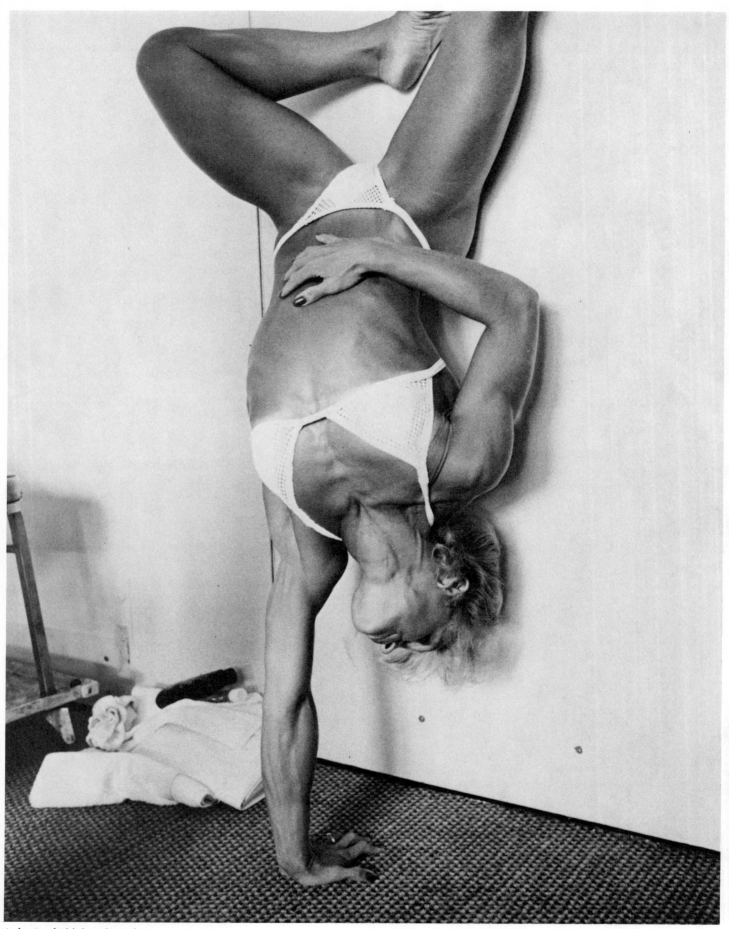

Auby Paulick's handstand

1

A small pale room on the mezzanine floor of the Philadelphia Sheraton Hotel, August 1980. The room is bare except for two small dumbbells, a barbell, and a big blue Corbin Gentry lat machine standing against one wall. At ten to one in the afternoon, Carolyn Cheshire, a willowy, ladylike bodybuilder and former model from Surrey, England, is alone in the room applying Man Tan to her shapely legs. She looks up as Patsy Chapman comes in. The two women smile at each other. Carolyn goes back to her legs. Patsy stands in the middle of the floor, staring at a wall, trying to shut out of her mind everything beyond it.

There is quite a bit out there to shut out. The Sheraton is hosting both the first Annual International Bodybuilding Convention and the first International Federation of Body Builders' Miss Olympia Competition this weekend, and the place is stuffed with old and new faces of bodybuilding. The traditional heads of state are all there—Arnold, Franco, Frank Zane, Joe and Ben Weider—along with a lot of others who go way back, like Ed Corney and Mike Katz, Ricky Wayne, Leroy Colbert, Oscar State, Dennis Tinnerino, Harold Poole, Armand Tanny and John Balik. But mixed in with those people, now that bodybuilding is big business, are hundreds of parvenus—television and print journalists, photographers in Bally loafers, equipment manufacturers, promoters, vitamin purveyors and gym owners—most of them selling or buying something, not just in the hotel's basement where a kind of bodybuilding trade show is going on, but in its lobby and elevators and conference rooms and suites as well; and most of them are here, specifically, to determine today and tonight at the prejudging and show of the Miss Olympia contest, the first really major women's bodybuilding competition ever held, if and how this newest and flashiest of bodybuilding's new products, this "lady's thing," is going to sell.

So there is an atmosphere of scrutiny in the hotel—not just the ordinary diffuse checking out of lats and triceps, but a very focused kind of commercial study.

An egg is being hatched here in the Philadelphia Sheraton this weekend, and the assembled representatives of the bodybusiness, old and new, are watching with particular attention, and with an eye to what's in it for them if the creature inside should happen to fly.

There is all of that for Patsy Chapman to put out of her mind in the pump-up room, forty minutes before the Miss Olympia prejudging. And there is something else as well. In a lot of people's books she is supposed to be the favorite here—she won last year's smaller and more tentative version of this contest, "The Best in the World"—and yet Patsy can't help noticing that some of the girls this year have *muscles,* not just quiet, well-toned muscles like her own, but veiny, chunky, stand-out ones, almost like the men have, and that makes her a little nervous. As the room begins to fill up with other contestants she realizes with increasing clarity that this is a different ball game from "The Best in the World." Patsy Chapman is black, twenty-one years old, a senior at Michigan State majoring in journalism. She has big calm eyes, a model's bones in her face, and a lovely body on which she has worked for five years, but as the room fills and the contestants disrobe, she becomes more and more sure that she will retire that body from competition after this contest, win or lose.

A pretty Danish girl named Anniqua Fors is doing dead-lifts, dressed in a caftan. Corinne Machado-Ching, a twenty-three-year-old dental assistant wearing a fuchsia bathing suit, is being oiled by her Oriental husband, and a disproportionate amount of room is being taken up by a tiny twenty-six-year-old nut-brown blonde named Auby Paulick from Birmingham, Michigan, who hogs the mirror, chuckling and flexing and jumping into gay, acrobatic poses. Scarcely dressed in a white bikini, Auby is one of the girls making Patsy Chapman wonder what exactly is going on here: Auby's midsection is not only hard but ridged, each chunk of the abdominals standing out cleanly, and her arms and back and upper chest are ropy with muscle.

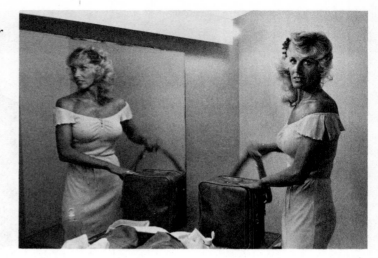

"When I got to college I got away from any strict routine as far as cheerleading training or practices or anything like that goes, and I went home one day and my Dad says, 'That's not the body I used to know.' I wasn't out of shape, believe me, but the muscle tone just wasn't all there. That's all he had to say. I immediately snapped and I went to a health club, a really nice spa with all kinds of equipment and weights, and I fell in love with the atmosphere."
—Rachel McLish

She does some one-arm handstands against the wall, then she prances over to the lat machine and poses on it for a photographer, taking half the eyes in the room with her. The other half are trained on Rachel McLish, who has just walked gravely in, wearing a halter top and a blue skirt, and who is, along with Patsy, the early favorite in this competition. Rachel is twenty-six and lives in Texas. A few months before, in her first contest, she won the U.S. Women's Bodybuilding Championship in Atlantic City. She has a long-waisted, well-defined, graceful body, nearly perfect legs, a few noticeable muscles here and there in her upper body, and a pretty, serious, big-eyed face. Most of all she has, like Auby Paulick, finish: a sort of polish to her body that comes from each part's bearing an elegant relationship to the whole. Very few bodybuilders, male or female, have it, and the ones who do will catch and hold your eye.

Pumping-up and oiling before a male prejudging is usually a somber affair. There are rarely any women present, rarely much conversation or any humor. Here in this little room in the Sheraton the mood is more open. Many of the women have their boyfriends or husbands with them to comfort and oil them. They chat and smile shyly, admire each other's posing suits, get out of each other's way. And the difference is carried into the prejudging itself. The men's prejudgings have a particular smell to them—a strong, acrid smell made up of nervousness, pride, sweat and baby oil. Almost as soon as the twenty-one women contestants file into the long, thin conference room full of standing official observers and press and take their places before the table of four men and three women judges, you can notice that the smell is interestingly different here—still acrid but sweeter and more tentative, as if it has in it some of the touching tractability and eagerness to please that soon become apparent in the contestants. Every one of these women *wants to win* this contest—not only for a piece of the ten-thousand-dollar total prize money, or for the trip to Venezuela that

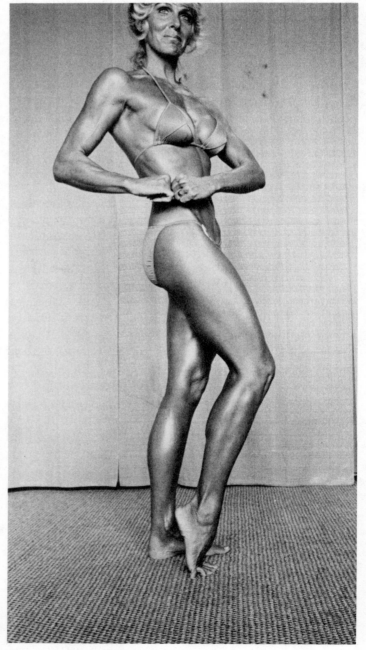

Georgia Miller-Fudge, 1980

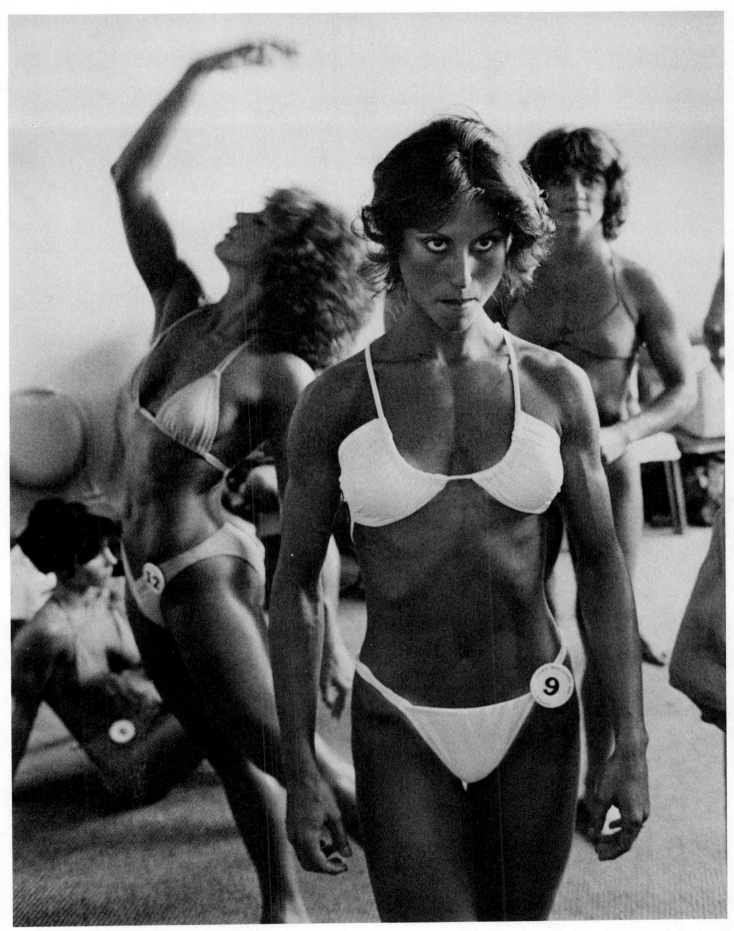

Pump-up room, Miss Olympia Competition, 1980

11

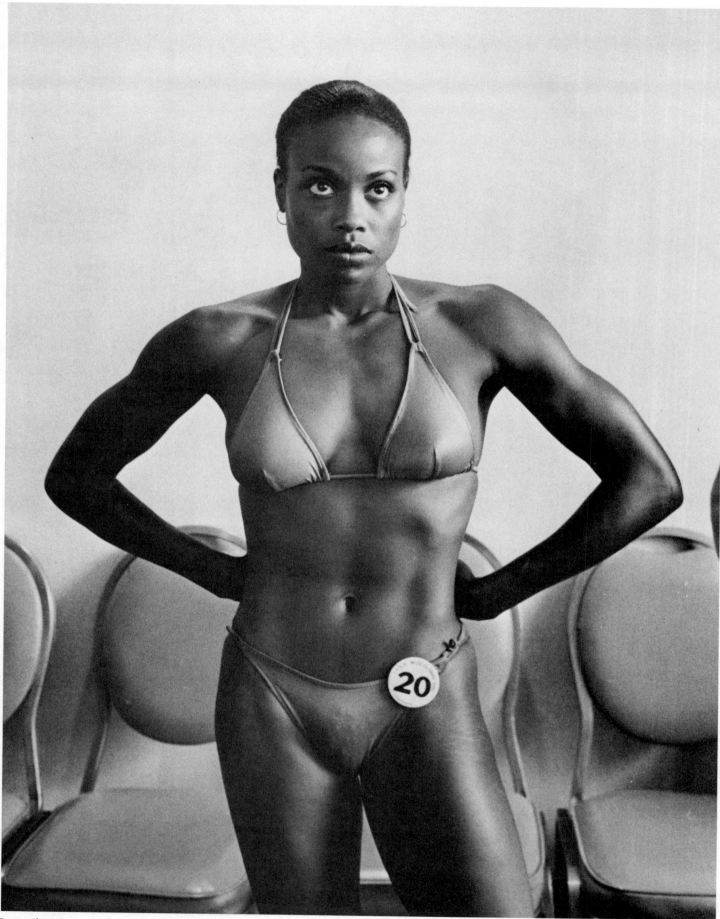

Patsy Chapman

will go to the top five finishers, but for the prestige and publicity that will accompany having won the first-ever Miss Olympia—but none of them knows exactly *how* to do it. All but five have won some title previously during the short two- or three-year period in which there have been titles to win in female bodybuilding, but the standards keep shifting and no one is sure what Christine Zane, Doris Barrilleaux, Harold Poole, Mike Katz, Dan Howard, Sven-Ole Thorsen, and Valerie Coe are looking for. The aesthetics of female bodybuilding are so new, and at this point so arbitrary, that these judges themselves are not in agreement about what to grade or how to grade it. Do they want big muscles? Symmetry? Definition? . . . The women peek at their evaluators, smiling hopefully, offering what they have.

April Nicotra and Lorie Johnston have bustlines and hips—nice traditional hourglass shapes; Patsy Chapman, Corinne Machado-Ching and Georgia Miller-Fudge, a handsome thirty-four-year-old gym owner from Florida, have these shapes too, but with more muscle; Lynn Conkwright and Stacey Bentley have athletic tomboy bodies, muscled like female gymnasts; Auby Paulick has no-nonsense *muscle*, as do Cammie Lusko, a stunt woman and strength-lifter from California and, to a lesser degree, Kyle Newman, Miss Long Island, a smoky, deep-voiced, straight-ahead brunette. And Rachel McLish? As the prejudging progresses it becomes evident that what Rachel has, in addition to finish, is enough of a number of things to provide a

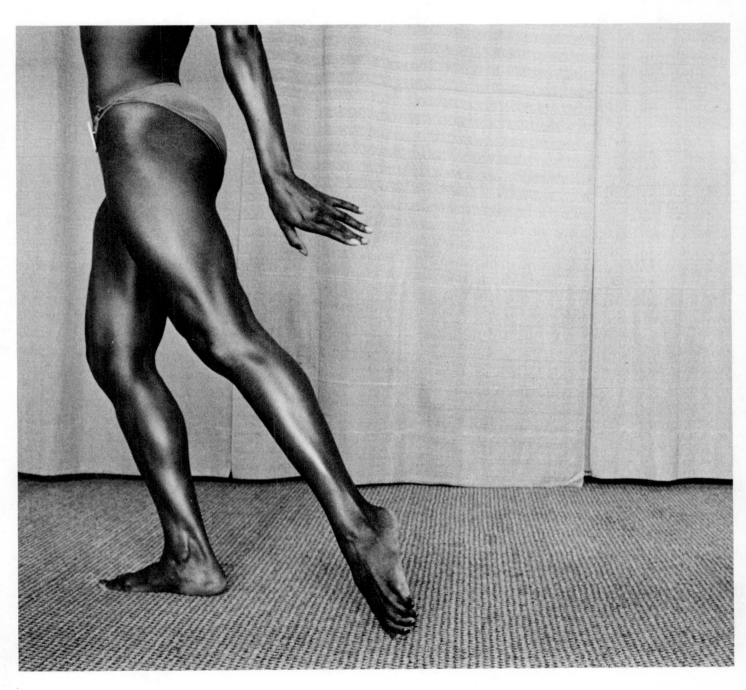

"When I pose I feel no sexual thing at all—I'm not out there being seductive."
—Lynn Conkwright

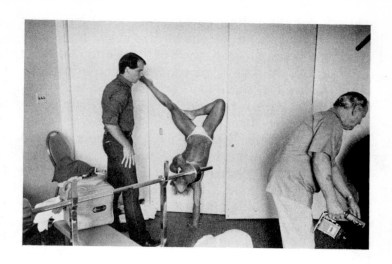

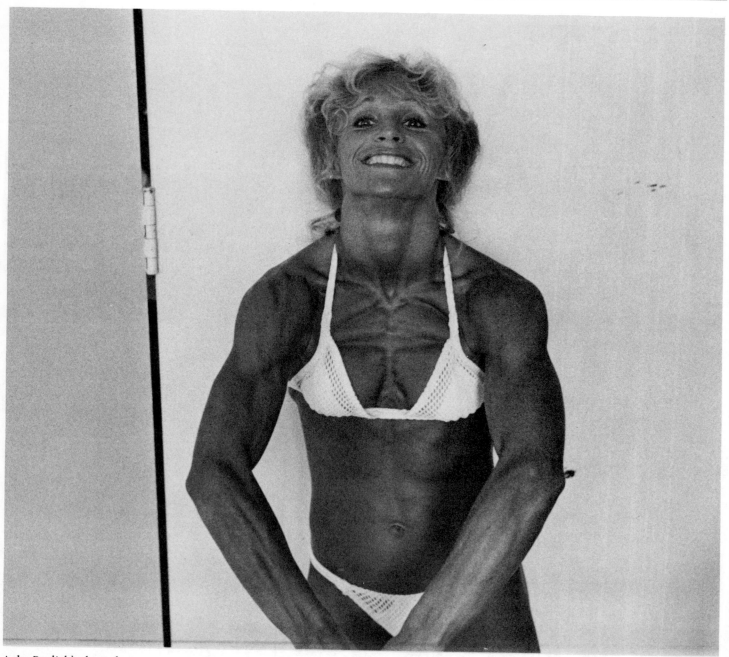

Auby Paulick's chest shot

compromise for any judge unsure himself, or herself, what exactly he or she is supposed to be looking for.

The prejudging consists of three rounds. In the first round each woman is observed relaxed from the front and rear and each side; in the second she demonstrates six compulsory poses designed to show all the muscle groups; and in the third, the round that will be duplicated at night for the presentation or performance of the contest, she has one minute to perform her own free routine of poses. The judging is done under the auspices of the International Federation of Body Builders' newly created Women's Committee, whose secretary, Cathy Gelfo, is in the room to make sure that all the competitors adhere to the committee's guidelines, guidelines which include such detailed

recommendations as this: "It should be remembered that this is a bodybuilding competition and over-reliance on elements outside the sport, that is, dance, gymnastics, etc., should not be favored. Attire should consist of a minimal two-pieced bathing suit, no shoes, a minimum of jewelry, no other ornamentation, tasteful makeup, with the hair preferably up or back if the hair is long."

The guidelines also encourage the competitors to pose gracefully in a nonmasculine way. And most of them do that—hitting sensual, curvilinear positions that are like frozen dance movements—but not all. In the second and third rounds a few girls, notably Cammie and Auby, throw out some real muscle poses, grabbers, "double-biceps" and "most musculars," the

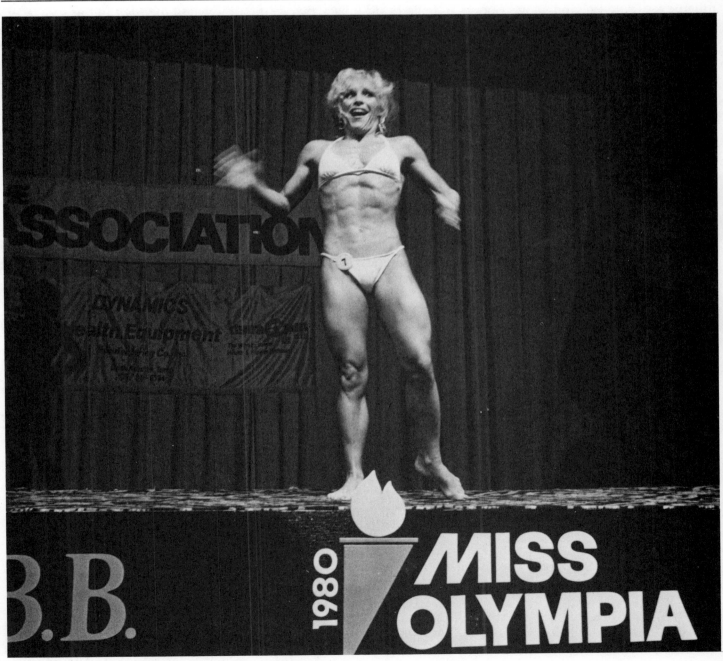

Auby Paulick, onstage. Miss Olympia Competition, 1980

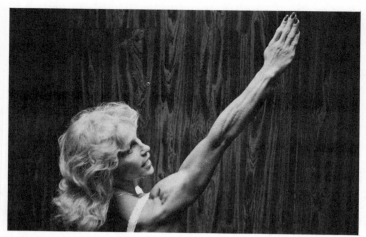
Auby Paulick

"Ever since I was in high school I was always real athletic, you know, my thighs were very big, just a very athletic type, my whole physique. And all the women then, it was the Twiggy look, being skinny and the blond hair and all this, and I always had to convince people, hey, you know to be healthy, it's not that bad. Why is it that men like the real skinny look?"
—Lynn Conkwright

fully flexed, vein-bulging showstoppers of male body-building, tensing for all they are worth, clenching their little fists (against guideline recommendations), and showing to an assembled group of people for perhaps the first time in history *real female muscle,* not just little curvy humps of hard flesh, but rippled, deline-ated, vein-splayed muscle in their thighs, their shoul-ders, their stomachs and chests, all the historically soft and comforting areas of a woman.

And all at once, right then, the cat was out of the bag. You could hear audible gasps in the room—and many, many more gasps, along with practically every other kind of human sound, that night in the ballroom of the hotel where fifteen hundred well-dressed folks, most of them new to female bodybuilding, gathered to dine and watch the show. To be honest, the show ruined a few appetites. Not Lorie Johnston or April Nicotra or Patsy Chapman, with their smooth, buxom, ladylike poses, which might as well have been an interesting extension of the bathing-suit competition of the Miss America contest. Those women and most of the others might have mildly riled a few male hormones and pointed out the aesthetic values of exercise to some out-of-shape women in the audience, but they didn't cause anyone, out of lust or horror or excitement, to turn away from their fruit cups and creamed chicken the way Cammie Lusko did when she popped out her "back double-biceps," or Auby Paulick did with her "crab" or her guidelines-foiling handstands and splits, or her delighted, self-absorbed, muscular prancing around on stage.

With Auby and Cammie, who made no effort to keep it in, the cat was, for good, out of the bag. The egg was hatched, and female bodybuilding, for better or worse, had arrived.

Ricky Wayne, for one, was horrified. Ricky is a stal-wart, an old pro who has been around bodybuilding —first as a world-class competitor and then as one of the sport's few good reporters—for years, from way back before the time when the *men* in the sport were taken to be something more than freaks. And yet at the prejudging he found himself "fighting everything within me that suggested what I was looking at was a scene from some weird science fiction movie," and deciding finally that "women simply were never meant to look like that."

Others were thrilled, turned on, inspired. Who knows what the bodybusinessmen thought? Though a number of them left Philadelphia at a dead run to capitalize on Rachel, who won the contest (but not so fast on Auby, who was its real star but came in second, and not at all on Cammie Lusko or Patsy Chapman, who didn't place), none of them was talking. The most interesting and maybe the most perceptive reaction came from Frank Zane. Better than practically anyone there that weekend, Frank understands bodybuilding. He was a Mr. Universe before Arnold Schwarzenegger arrived in this country and a Mr. Olympia three times after Arnold retired for the first time. But watching the show that night there was a slightly mystified expres-sion on his face. This much at least about what had been hatched this weekend in Philadelphia was clear to Frank Zane: it had no precedent.

"You familiar with Carl Jung?" he asked someone next to him during the show.

"Yeah."

"Well, I don't think there's an archetype for this."

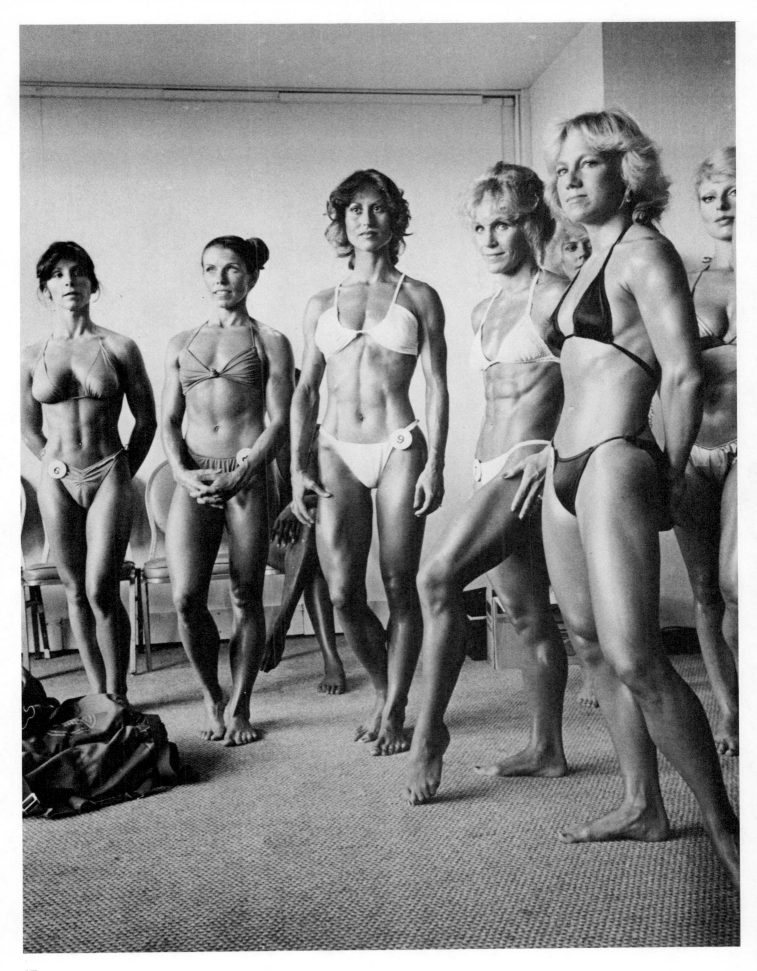

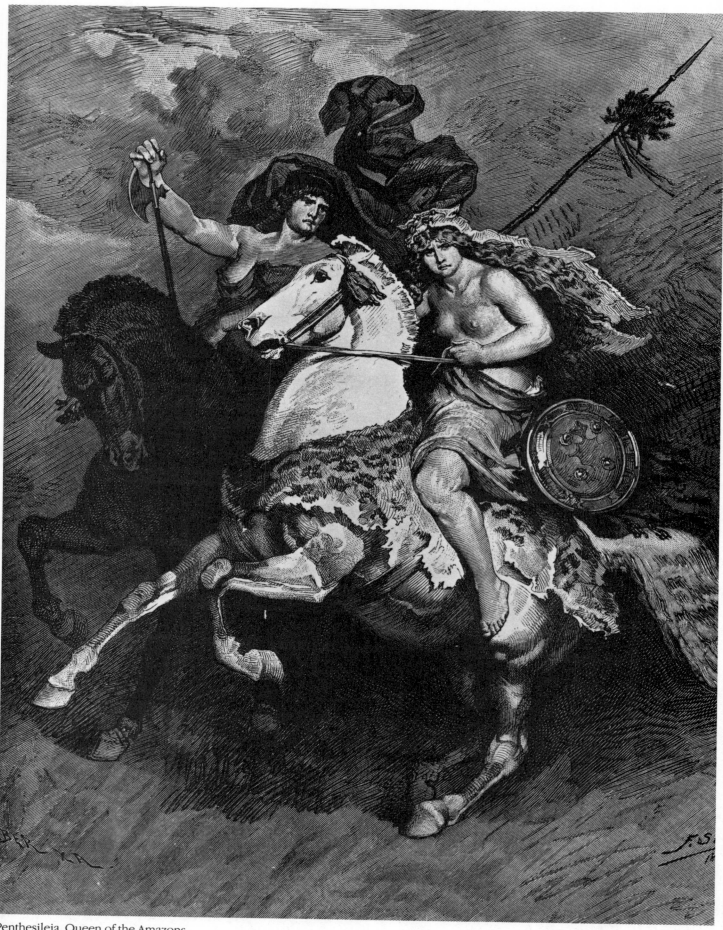

Penthesileia, Queen of the Amazons

(Bettmann Archive)

2

The question is, where in the world, in the history of the world, did women with muscles come from? The answer is, not many places. Though standards of beauty for women have historically varied more often and more radically than those for men, it is difficult to find muscular women celebrated or even recorded anywhere in written or visual history, including mythology.

There are, of course, the Amazons—the probably mythic race of warrior women supposed by Herodotus to have lived during the thirteenth century B.C. on the north coast of Asia Minor and to have battled various Greek heroes, including Achilles, Priam, Hercules and Theseus. Also in myth we find Diana, the strong-limbed goddess of the moon and the hunt, protectress of women, identified by the Romans with the Greeks' Artemis; and Atalanta, the Greek devotee of Artemis, who was suckled by a she-bear, who outwrestled Peleus, the father of Achilles, and could outrun any man in Greece. Folk tales and myths of women warriors are also found, scattered and thin, in China, India, Africa, the Arab countries, the British Isles, Scandinavia, among the Makurap people of Brazil, and the Eskimos of Kodiak Island. There is Macha, the fierce warrior goddess of the Celts, Brynhild of the *Volsunga Saga*, Egee of Libya, Penthesileia of North Africa and Eurpyle of the Near East, leader of a women's expedition against Babylonia in the seventeenth century B.C. . . . And that pretty well covers it.

Most of these women are not portrayed, either verbally or visually, as being particularly strong or well muscled, but simply as superhuman. An occasional statue of Diana will show slightly bulging deltoids, natural to an archer; one of the Ephesus Amazons has beautifully muscled calves and some triceps. But on the whole these make-believe heroines were described, painted and sculpted in conventional physical terms.

So far as real-life history is concerned, probably the first record of strong, overtly athletic women in West-

ern culture is found in the Minoan Toreras, statues of wasp-waisted, big-thighed female bull-leapers from Minoan Crete, a gay, extroverted society which reached its zenith around 1400 B.C. After that there was Greece, or more specifically, Sparta. Athens and the other city-states of classical Greece did not believe in women exercising; they believed in converting them into mothers early and keeping them indoors. In Athens, perhaps by way of discouraging female athletic energy, girls in a household were allowed less than half the food allotted their brothers. But Spartan girls were as well nourished as the boys and encouraged by the Spartan regime—developed by the lawgiver Lycurgus in the seventh century B.C.—to exercise at racing, throwing the quoit and javelin and even at wrestling. The Athenians were shocked by this practice and by the fact that Spartan women exercised either in the nude or wearing only the Doric *peplos* tunic, which revealed their thighs. The poet Ibycus referred to these women as nymphomaniacs, and Euripides grumbles in his "Andromache" that "they gad abroad with young men with naked thighs. And with clothes discarded they race with them, wrestle with them. Intolerable!" But Plutarch insists that there was no wantonness in the *déshabille* of Spartan women, only pride and pleasure in the beauty and health of the body which their laws, uniquely in ancient culture, allowed them to develop. Cynisca, a tall, hefty daughter of one of the royal houses of Sparta, even took sufficient advantage of those laws to become the first woman victor at Olympia, in the *quadriga* chariot race, at the beginning of the fourth century B.C.

We know that some upper-class Roman women exercised, and there is this hint in Juvenal that a few might have even lifted weights in some formal way: "It is at night that she goes to the baths, at night that she gives orders for her oil flasks and other impedimenta to be taken there; she loves to sweat among the noise and bustle. When her arms fall to her sides, worn out by the heavy weights, the skillful masseur presses his fingers into her body, and makes her bottom resound with his loud smack." But after the Romans, from about the first century B.C. onward, the muscular woman virtually disappears in history.

When something exists as an archetype, it is played as theme and variation over and over again down the centuries, cropping up in culture after culture with minor stylistic alterations but essentially the same as when it was first perceived. Nowhere is this principle more evident than in art history, the visual record of our archetypal preoccupations—and the history of art is practically as barren of truly muscular women as it is of, say, men with breasts. The shape to which the female body tends to return throughout the entire history of art—its archetypal shape—is one which em-

phasizes its biological functions, those life-begetting and sustaining functions which since the very earliest cultures have been most often suggested by a softly curved cello shape, what Sir Kenneth Clark calls "an oval, surmounted by two spheres." Since prehistory it has occurred to very few artists to overlay that shape, with all its conscious and subconscious allure, with biologically irrelevant muscle—and if you should doubt that this is true, a look through Clark's definitive study of the human body in art, *The Nude,* might prove instructive. There, among the hundreds of plates of women painted and sculpted, from prehistoric Cycladic dolls on up through Picasso bathers, you will find only these depicted with anything more than normal female musculature: a bronze Venus by the six-

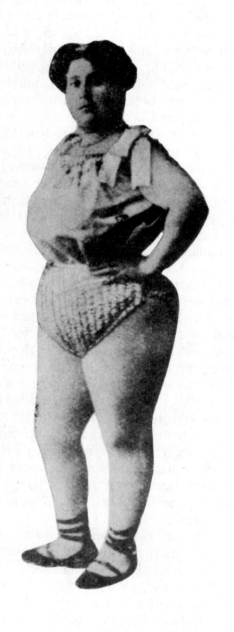

Mme. Montagna

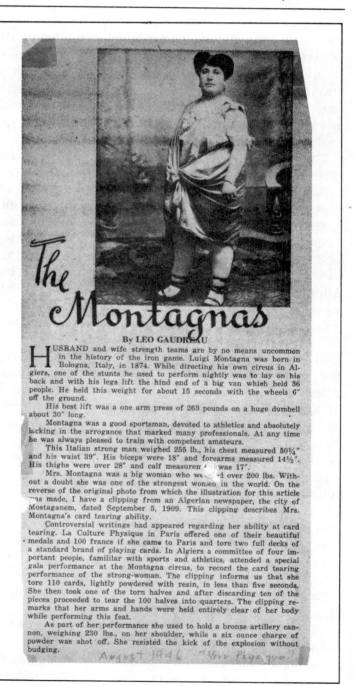

The Montagnas

By LEO GAUDREAU

HUSBAND and wife strength teams are by no means uncommon in the history of the iron game. Luigi Montagna was born in Bologna, Italy, in 1874. While directing his own circus in Algiers, one of the stunts he used to perform nightly was to lay on his back and with his legs lift the hind end of a big van which held 36 people. He held this weight for about 15 seconds with the wheels 6" off the ground.

His best lift was a one arm press of 263 pounds on a huge dumbell about 30" long.

Montagna was a good sportsman, devoted to athletics and absolutely lacking in the arrogance that marked many professionals. At any time he was always pleased to train with competent amateurs.

This Italian strong man weighed 255 lb., his chest measured 50¼" and his waist 39". His biceps were 18" and forearms measured 14½". His thighs were over 28" and calf measurem   was 17".

Mrs. Montagna was a big woman who we   d over 200 lbs. Without a doubt she was one of the strongest women in the world. On the reverse of the original photo from which the illustration for this article   as made, I have a clipping from an Algerian newspaper, the city of Mostaganem, dated September 5, 1909. This clipping describes Mrs. Montagna's card tearing ability.

Controversial writings had appeared regarding her ability at card tearing. La Culture Physique in Paris offered one of their beautiful medals and 100 francs if she came to Paris and tore two full decks of a standard brand of playing cards. In Algiers a committee of four important people, familiar with sports and athletics, attended a special gala performance at the Montagna circus, to record the card tearing performance of the strong-woman. The clipping informs us that she tore 110 cards, lightly powdered with resin, in less than five seconds. She then took one of the torn halves and after discarding ten of the pieces proceeded to tear the 100 halves into quarters. The clipping remarks that her arms and hands were held entirely clear of her body while performing this feat.

As part of her performance she used to hold a bronze artillery cannon, weighing 230 lbs., on her shoulder, while a six ounce charge of powder was shot off. She resisted the kick of the explosion without budging.

August 1946 "Your Phys qua"

teenth-century Florentine Ammanati, a long-waisted, beautiful-legged and seductive statue that Rachel McLish might have posed for; a strange-to-grotesque engraving of Vitruvian woman, also done in the sixteenth century, by Dürer; a drawing of girls wrestling by the nineteenth-century painter Delacroix; and, again from the sixteenth century, the most muscular women in all of art history, Michelangelo's statues of Dawn and Night, the studies for which were drawn from male models.

Now even these are *modestly* muscular women, you understand, with most of their strength represented in their haunches and buttocks. *Nowhere* in the history of female depiction can you find a back like Cammie Lusko's, or a midsection like Auby Paulick's.

In written history, as mentioned, women with any kind of muscles at all, physically strong, athletically capable women, virtually disappear after the first century B.C., and they do not emerge again until the late nineteenth century. To be sure there were women during that interim who have been recorded as accomplishing impressive physical deeds, women in the Amazon mode—Joan of Arc, for example; and Hannah Dustin, the seventeenth-century American who killed and scalped nine Indians who had kidnapped herself and her baby; and Jeanne Laisné, the fifteenth-century French heroine who repelled a Burgundian attack on the village of Beauvais with a hatchet—but, like the Amazons, these women historically were noted not so much for their strength or physical impressiveness per

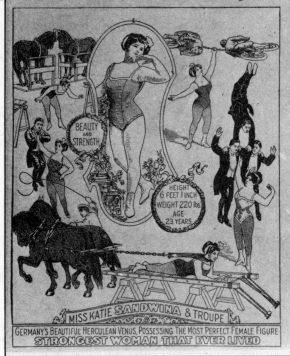

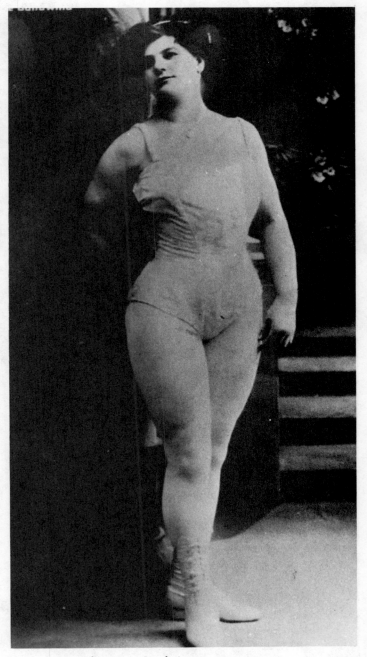

The Lady Hercules: Katie Sandwina

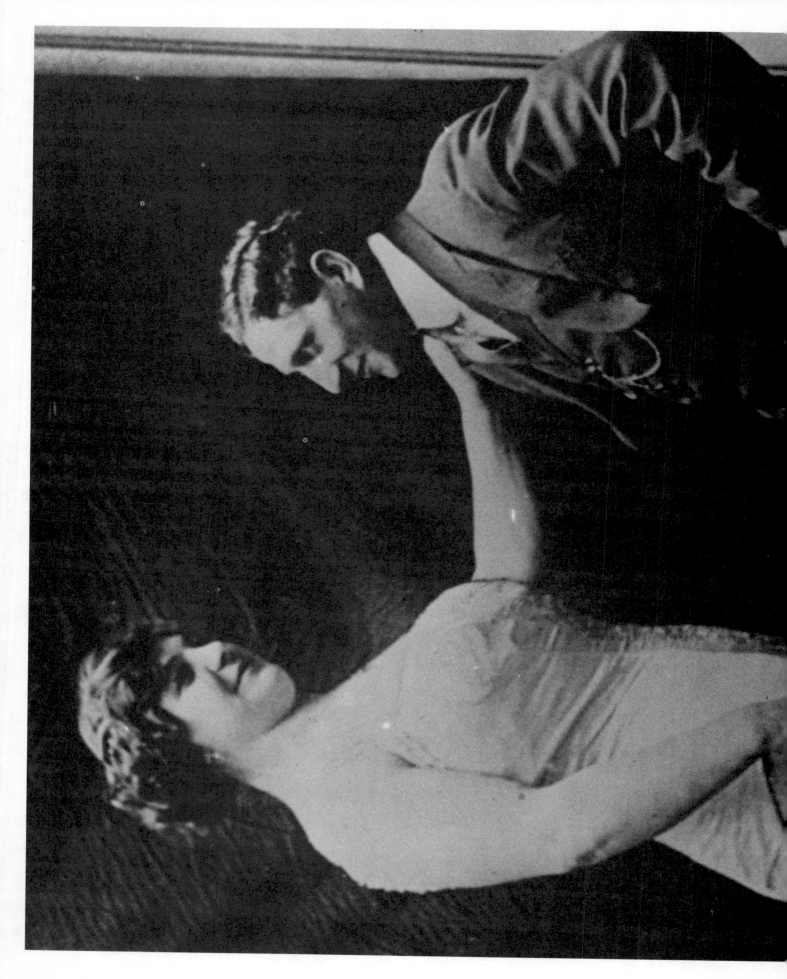

Kate Brumbach
(Sandwina)

se as for their willingness to use themselves physically in ways more traditionally masculine than feminine. If women bodybuilders have no archetype in history, they have in these Amazon-like accomplishers, these female doers of male deeds, an indirect precedence; and with the emergence in the late nineteenth century of the performing strongwoman they acquired a direct one as well.

In England there was "Vulcana," née Kate Roberts; in Italy there was "Miss Ella," a strongwoman with the Sciavoni Troupe who could carry four men around the stage on her shoulders and hold two men over her head; in Canada there was Louise Armaindo, and Mme. Cloutier, and Flossie La Branche; and in America there was "Minerva," Mrs. Josephine Blatt of Hoboken, New Jersey, who in the 1890s, at six feet and two hundred thirty pounds, performed a harness-lift of twenty-three men weighing, with the platform and chains, 3,564 pounds, and was proclaimed by *The Police Gazette* to be the strongest woman in the world.

But that title probably belonged to the most famous strongwoman of them all, the fabulous Austrian, Katie Sandwina. Born in 1884 to a circus family, Katie was twisting steel bars in a vaudeville act by the time she was a teenager. In her prime she stood six feet one and weighed two hundred nine pounds which was distributed over a handsome figure. During her years as a star with the Barnum and Bailey Circus she is said to have indulged a fondness for the spectacular by carrying her husband around over her head with one

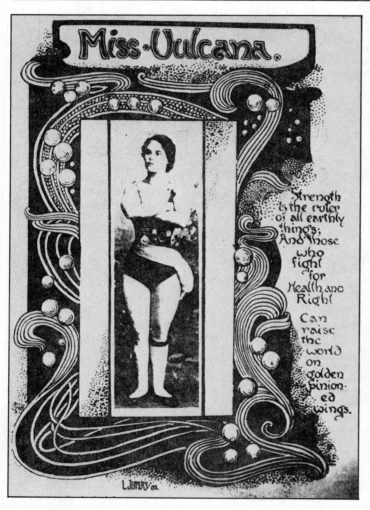

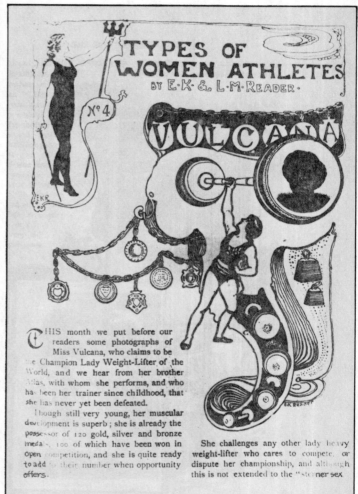

hand, supporting half-ton cannons on her back, and serving as the support for a bridge while forty men and horses trotted over it, as well as by legitimately and regularly jerking more than two hundred eighty pounds overhead.

Katie and Minerva and Flossie and Vulcana and the rest were a short-lived phenomenon. Though Katie continued to perform until the 1940s, it was only during the final two decades of the last century and the first two of this one that there was any real audience for strongwomen, and even then there was not much of one. But short-lived or not, the phenomenon was the real thing—women with muscles, that historical oddity—and though those women did not demonstrate their muscles as such but rather the strength of them, they are the closest thing in history to true precursors of modern women bodybuilders. Women bodybuilders may not have in those strongwomen—or in the Minoan Toreras, the Amazons, or the Spartan women—the archetype that Frank Zane found wanting, but they have at least a group of stout cousins to make the centuries feel less lonely.

The second question is, why now? Why and how did women's bodybuilding occur now, springing nearly full-blown out of the late 1970s? At least one answer is that nothing of much importance happens in spite of fashion. Women's bodybuilding could not have occurred in the fifties when women did not sweat, or in the sixties when practically every female in the world

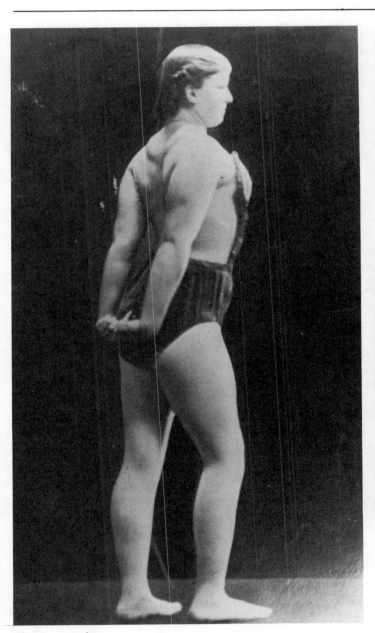

The Great Vulcana

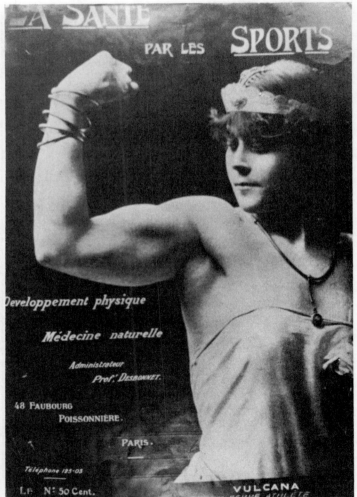

LA SANTÉ PAR LES SPORTS

Developpement physique

Médecine naturelle

Administrateur
Prof.ʳ DESBONNET.

48 FAUBOURG
POISSONNIÈRE.

PARIS.

Téléphone 125-03

Lᴿ Nᵒ 50 Cent.

VULCANA
FEMME ATHLÈTE

wanted to look like Twiggy—it had to wait for the last few years of the seventies when ripening feminism and a worldwide craze for fitness combined to produce a fashion that all but forced it to occur. That fashion, like all fashions a clear broth drained from a rich social stew, consisted of the ERA, women jet pilots and jockeys and executives and football players; jogging; halter tops, nylon shorts and New Balance running shoes; diet and exercise books; Kenneth Cooper, Arnold Schwarzenegger, James Fixx, Richard Simmons; sprouts, yogurt, yoga, herb teas, racquet ball, triathlons, biomechanics, fun-runs, "pumping iron," "staying hard." . . . The broth was clear and strong and good for you. It was Cheryl Tiegs wearing shorts and a muscular smile, Margaux Hemingway with her hair wet,

Brooke Shields naked on an island in a movie and then describing to a magazine her favorite stomach exercises, Jane Fonda stretching and standing up for her rights. And within this context women's bodybuilding fairly had to happen.

Though it can be said to have happened all at once, to have actually hatched and wobbled into the world at the Miss Olympia contest in Philadelphia in 1980, it was at least a decade in gestation. Its parents were male bodybuilding competitions and the second-rate beauty contests that were occasionally staged at some of the male competitions between weight-classes. The London Mr. Universe competition had such a contest, and so did the Mr. Olympia at the Brooklyn Academy of Music when George Butler and I first started going

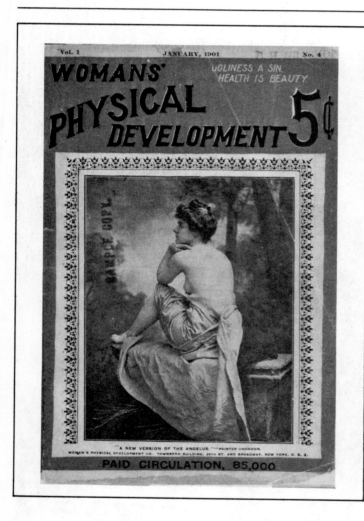

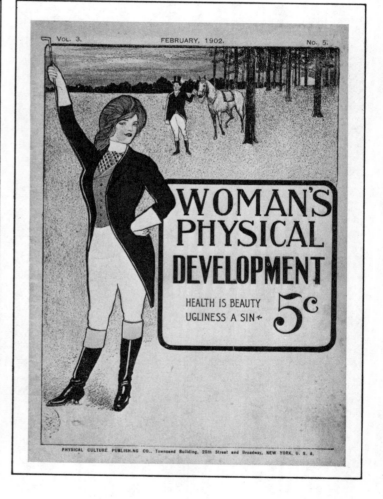

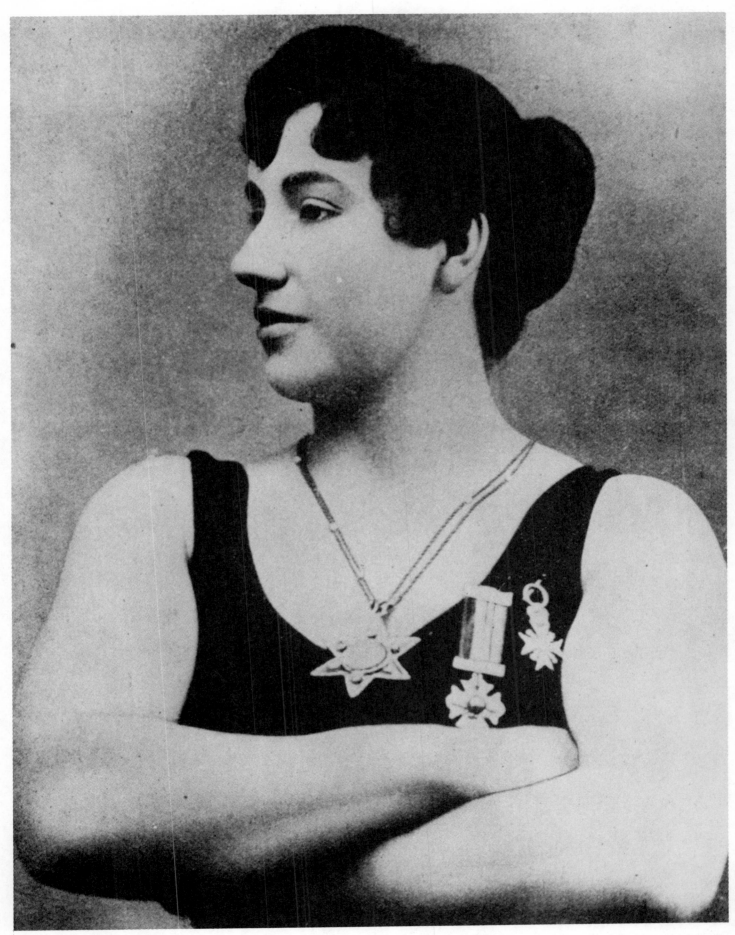

19th-century strongwoman

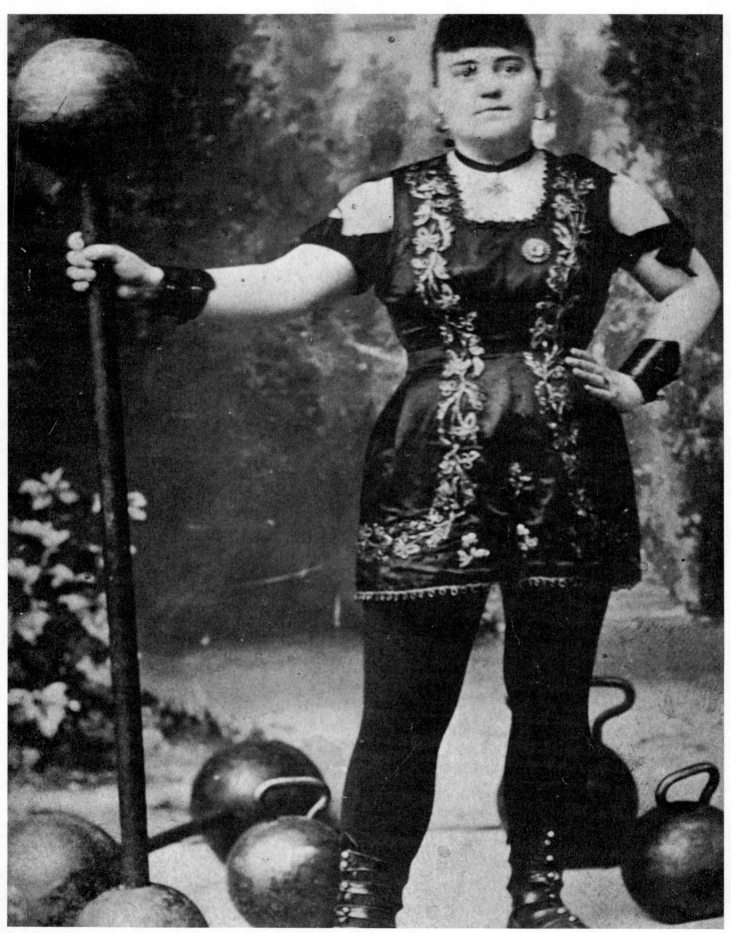

"Madame Minerva" with 185-pound barbell

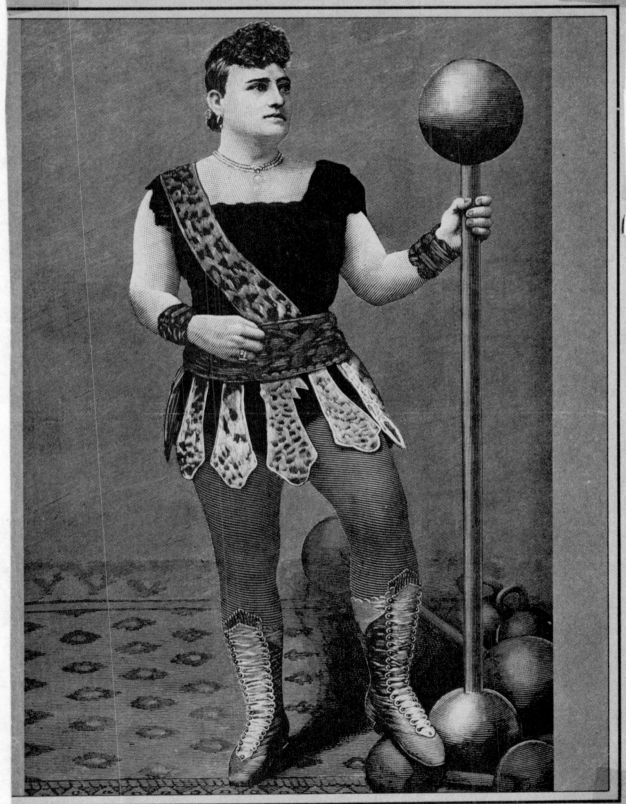

"MINERVA"

Gazette Champion Strong Woman of the World Who Defeated All Opponents and accomplished astounding feats.

(Reproduced from the original Police Gazette woodcut—1893)

POLICE GAZETTE, JULY, 1961

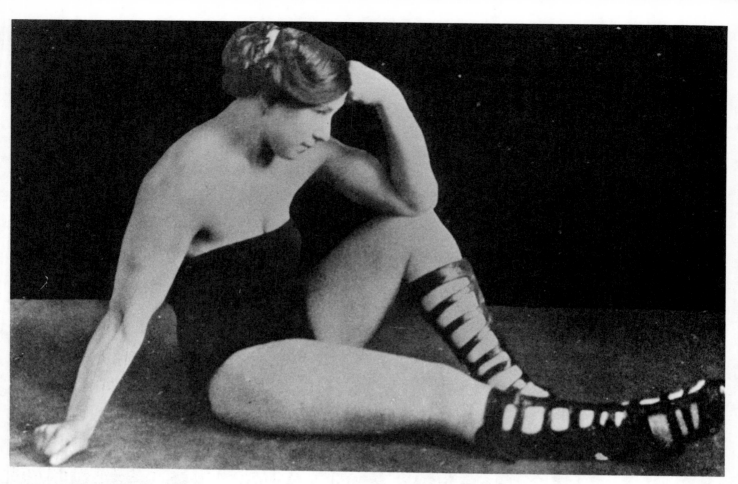

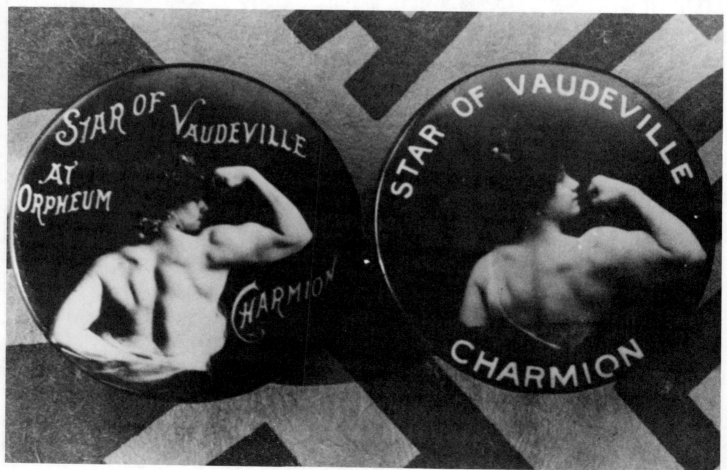

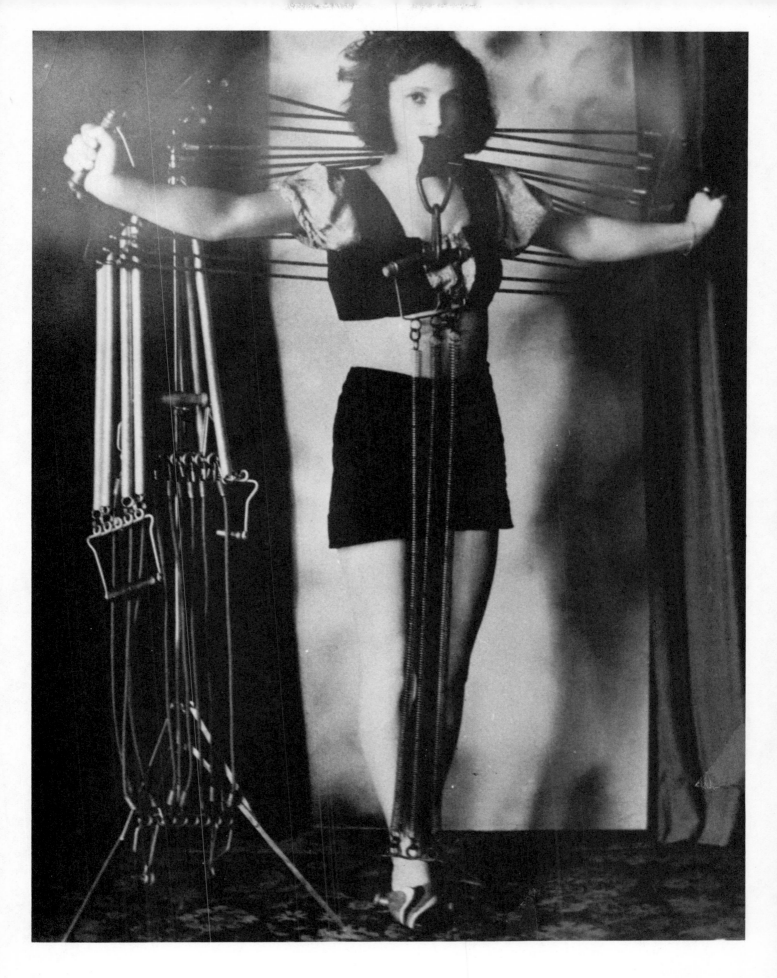

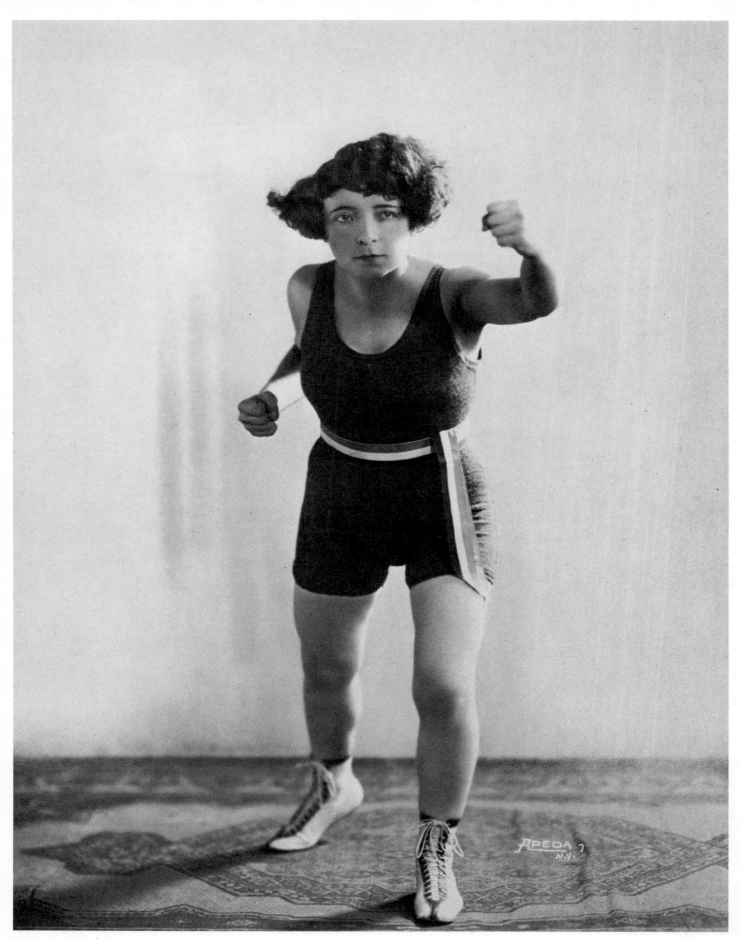

Jeanne Lamar, champion female boxer

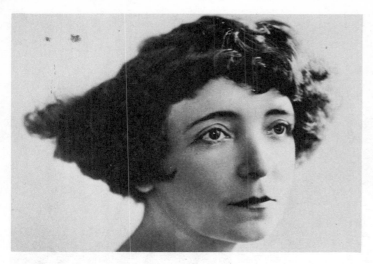

to bodybuilding competitions in the early seventies. The contest at the Mr. Olympia was called the Miss Americana. It was your typical bikini and stiletto-heel affair, where the women would come gyrating out to old bump-and-grind music, showing a lot of bosom and fingernails like red daggers. But once in a while, hyped by all the veiny male muscle backstage and the truly rabid crowds at the Academy, one of the contestants would throw a shy little muscle pose into her routine—flex a biceps, say—and it would *bring down the house*.

Then muscles got famous on the person of Arnold Schwarzenegger—largely through the movie *Stay Hungry* and the book and movie versions of *Pumping Iron*—and then, finally, legitimate. In the mid-seven-

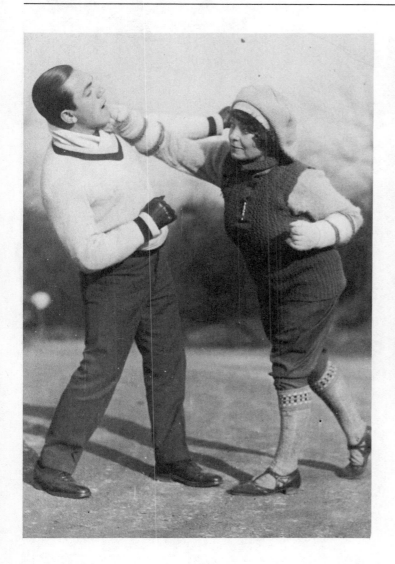

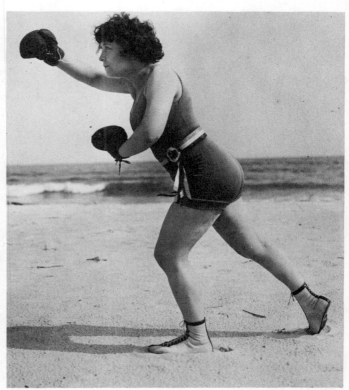

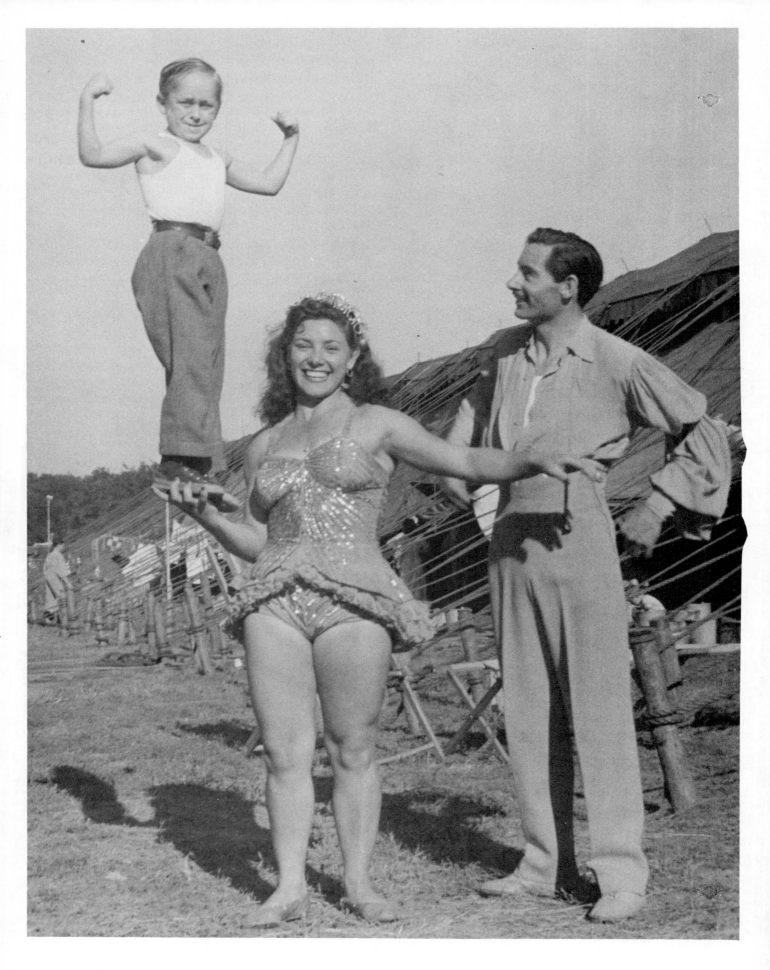

ties thousands of ordinary men started working out, not just for better health but to *look* better, and hard, developed male bodies became fashionable. You could see it anywhere you looked in this country, in movies and television, in magazines and advertisements, and everywhere on the street. Women, of course, were watching. They had recently learned that they could do what they wanted with themselves, and what more and more of them came to want in the mid- to late seventies was less fat on their thighs, less hip and droopy backs of the arm, and more of the ornamental fitness they saw being worn everywhere by men. Too, there were a lot of tomboys around, women who liked to sweat, after centuries of being told they shouldn't, and who were willing and eager to train

hard to do it. Women convinced themselves during the seventies that they weren't all that delicate after all, and that they owned their own bodies. To improve their figures or their health, or out of boredom or to prove to men that they could do it, or just to sweat and enjoy it, they took, in astounding numbers, to jogging in the park and cycling and aerobics and jazzercise, and more than a few of them took to *pumping iron*.

Doris Barrilleaux was out there waiting for them. Doris is fifty-one now, a tanned, startlingly fit grandmother from Florida. She began training with weights in the late fifties after having had four children, and the training stuck. She took up physique photography and was irked in the seventies that the only legitimate place for a woman in physique competitions was up

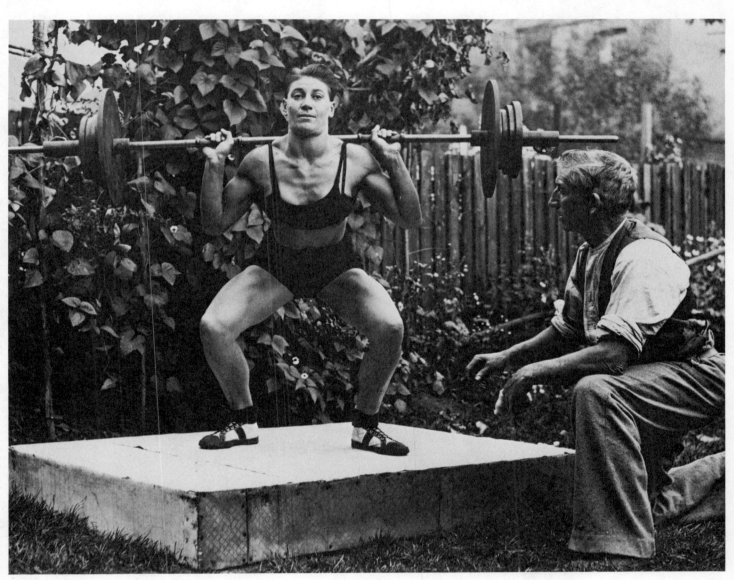

England, 1940s

Circus performers, 1930s

35

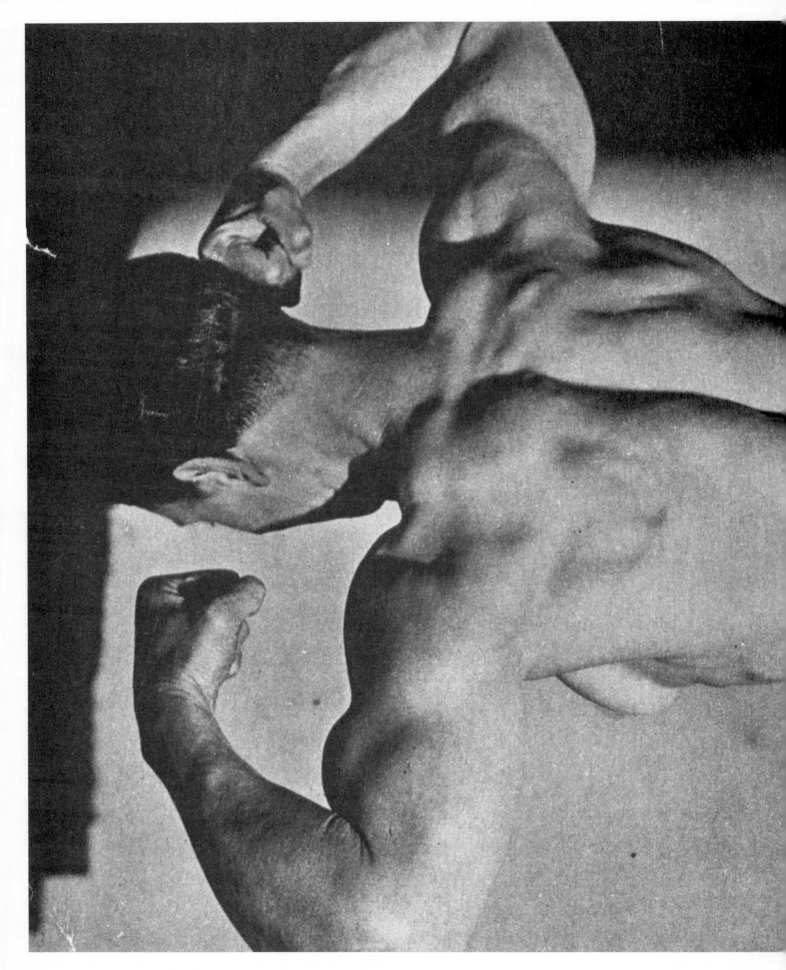

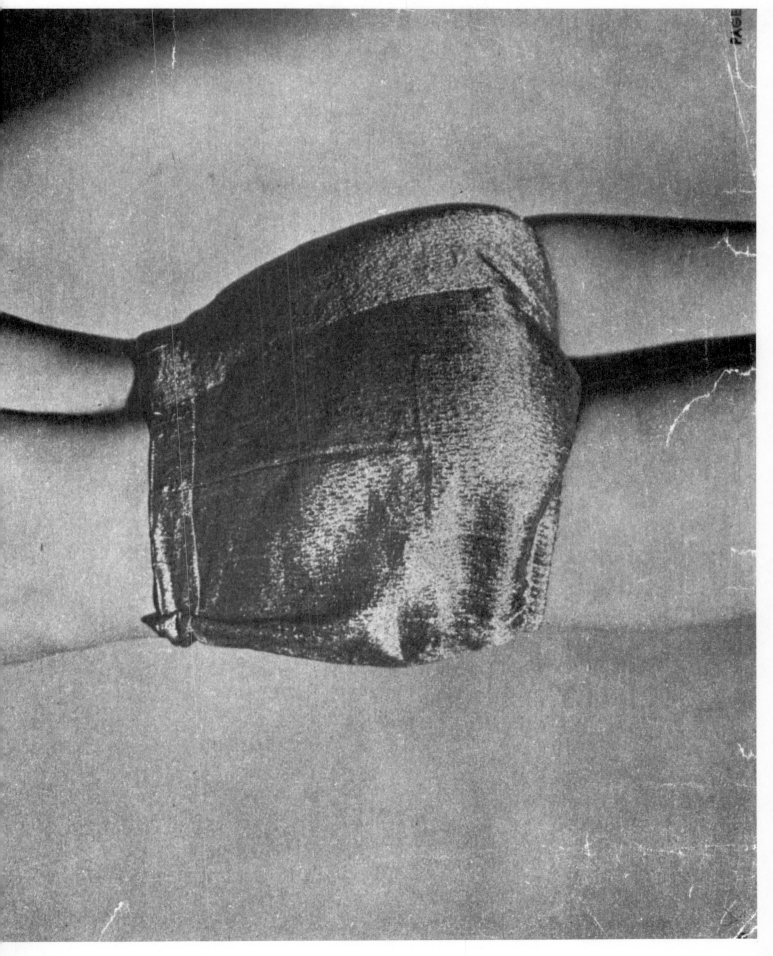

37

Her fabulous back

"Bodybuilding is definitely an evolution of the concept of femininity. Musculature is something that's very animal, but it's in no way a contradiction with femininity. Why should muscles be considered masculine? It's redefining the whole idea of femininity. You don't have to be soft, you don't have to be weak. You can be strong, you can be muscular —you can make that visual statement and at the same time be feminine. I think I have a very feminine body. I think of myself entirely as a woman."
—Lisa Lyon

on the stage handing out trophies to the men. She and some of her friends in Florida began to talk about the possibility of women's contests. Doris said to herself, "Women can do things now that they never could. They can be airline pilots; they can be telephone linemen; they can be tugboat captains; they can be anything they want. Why can't they be competitive bodybuilders?" In 1978 she read about a women's contest being held in Canton, Ohio. She was forty-seven. She trained hard and put together a routine to the song "I Am Woman." The contest, she says, was a mess. Two months later a man named George Snyder from Warrington, Pennsylvania, put on another contest, the first forerunner to the Miss Olympia competitions which Snyder later would develop and promote.

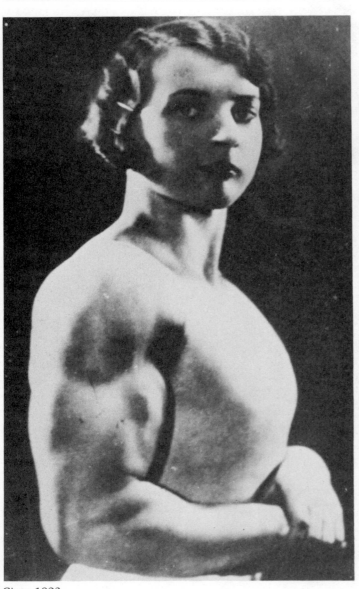

Circa 1923

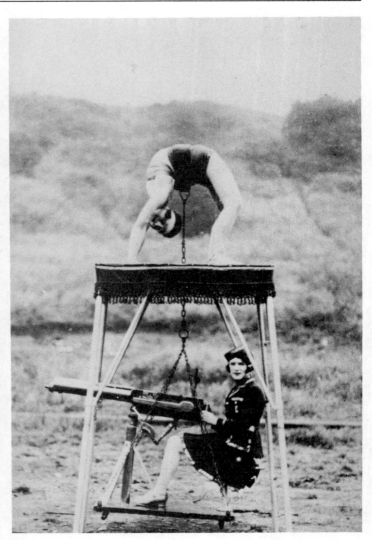

Target practice

"His was billed as a bodybuilding contest, but everyone knew it was a beauty contest," says Doris. "There were only two of us who did bodybuilding poses and that was a thirty-eight-year-old woman and myself. The rest were models that twirled and did the modeling poses, and the hoochy-koochy burlesque types who did their shaking at the audience.... At that contest Frank Zane took me aside and he says, 'Doris, the world's not ready for women bodybuilding.' And that did it. I had to show them that it was.... So I went home and there was a contest the next week or so, a men's contest. I said, 'Would you like a guest poser?' They said, 'Oh yeah, yeah.' No one had ever seen a lady guest poser. So I did it at the Southeastern, or whatever it was, there in Tampa, and after that the girls came up to me and said, 'Why can't we have something for women? Why don't we start something for women?' And so then the Superior Physique Association was formed."

SPA, it is called, and it was the first women's bodybuilding organization. Doris founded it in 1978, and in the next year began to publish the *SPA News,* a chatty, strongly editorial little newsletter devoted entirely to female bodybuilding. Through it and the other busy machinations of SPA, Doris became one of the two primary midwives for the birth of women's bodybuilding.

The other was a bright, articulate, good-looking UCLA cum laude graduate in anthropology named Lisa

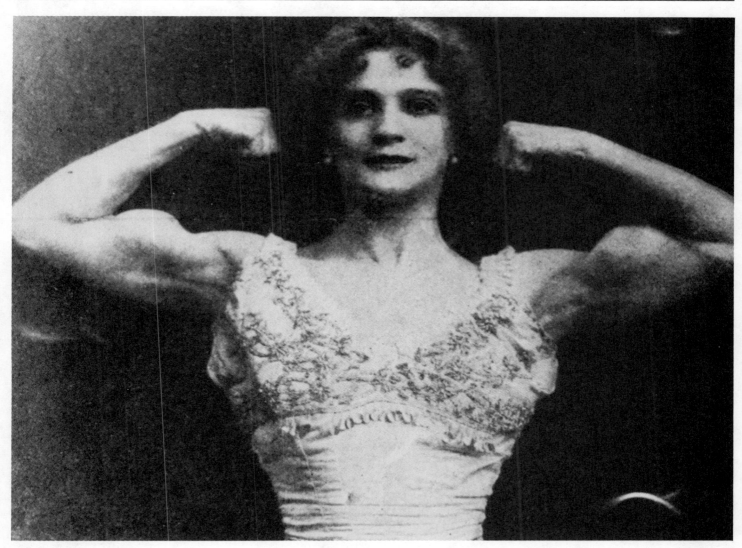

Mlle Ani

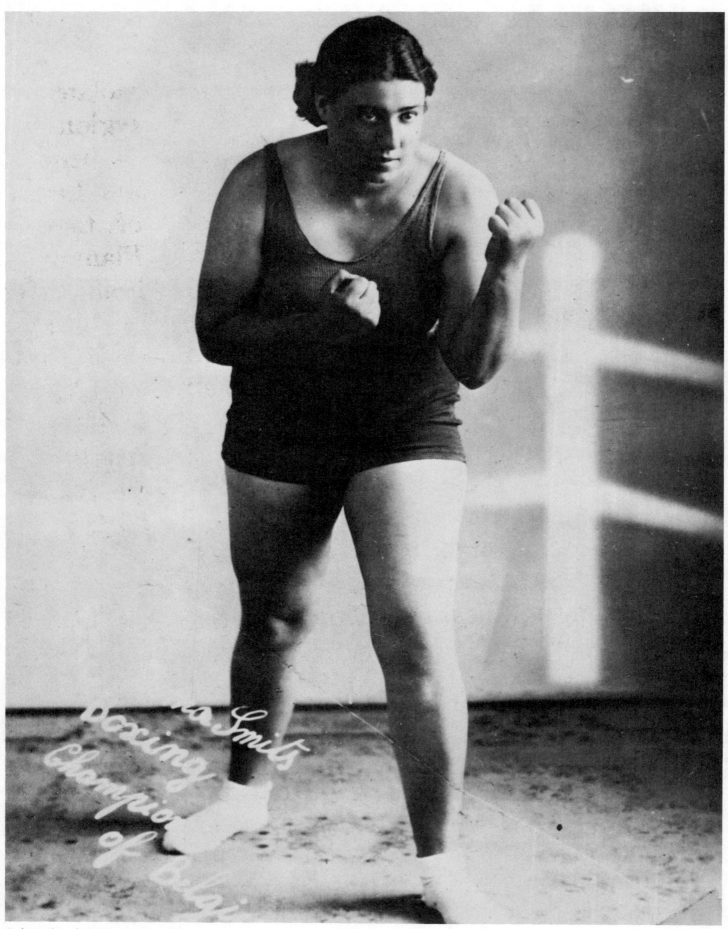

Belgian female boxing champion

Lyon. Lisa Lyon got into bodybuilding in California in the mid-seventies by way of kendo, a Japanese martïal art, and by way of Arnold Schwarzenegger, whom she met when she began to train with weights at Gold's Gym, at first just to get stronger for kendo. After a while at Gold's, encouraged by Arnold, she began to see that she "was creating a new aesthetic and a new standard of beauty—a high-tech body." And in 1979 she entered that body in the first World Women's Bodybuilding Championship, another of the beauty-contest, birthing-effort competitions like the ones Doris was entering, and won it.

Lisa Lyon had then and has now a taut, sleek, feminine body, a body no one could find offensive, which together with her pretty face, her articulateness and an

"Women can be airline pilots, they can be telephone linemen, they can be tugboat captains, they can be anything they want. So why can't they be bodybuilders?"
—Doris Barrilleaux

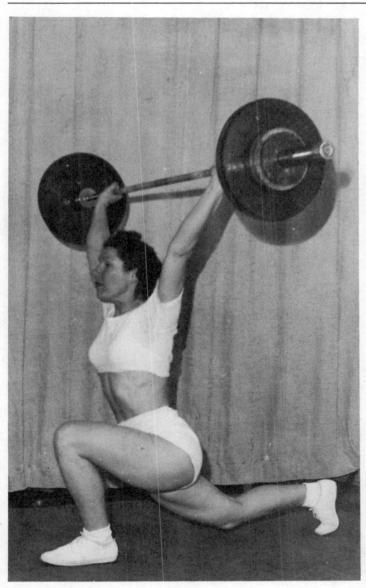 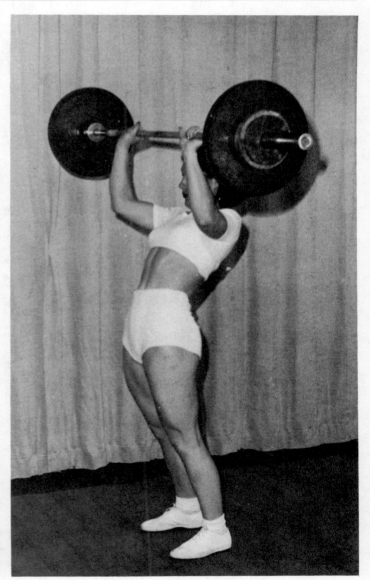

Clean and jerk, 1950s

impressive dedication to self-promotion, made her for a while not only, with Doris, women's bodybuilding's chief spokeswoman, but—even before the sport was really born—its only real media star. For about a year and a half during the late seventies she was in newspapers and magazines, and on television and radio shows, saying nicely phrased things about herself and muscles on women, and believing, as she told a *Washington Post* reporter, that "a pretty girl can sell anything." She posed for *Playboy*. She published a book. She helped to set up the National Physique Committee and the Women's Committee of the International Federation of Body Builders (the big daddy of the male organizations). She worked with women at Gold's Gym and helped to organize competitions and to draft the rules governing them. But she did not compete again.

By 1980 there were women around with a lot more muscle than Lisa Lyon had or wanted to have. "Bodybuilding," she told a magazine, "is definitely an evolution of the concept of femininity. Musculature is something that's very animal, but it's in no way a contradiction with femininity. Why should muscles be considered masculine? It's redefining the whole idea of femininity. You don't have to be soft, you don't have to be weak. You can be strong, you can be muscular—you can make that visual statement and at the same time be feminine. I think I have a very feminine body. I think of myself entirely as a woman." It might have been that she realized her body was entirely *too* feminine for what was coming or simply that she burned out, but for whatever reason, she retired, first from

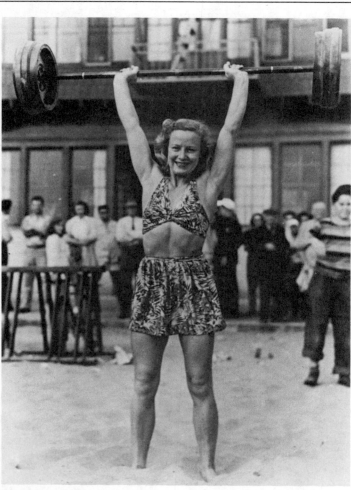

Ladies' Muscle Beach

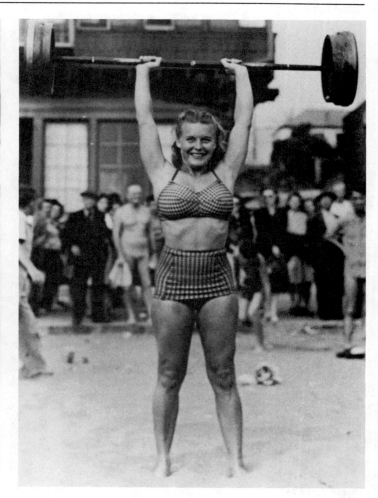

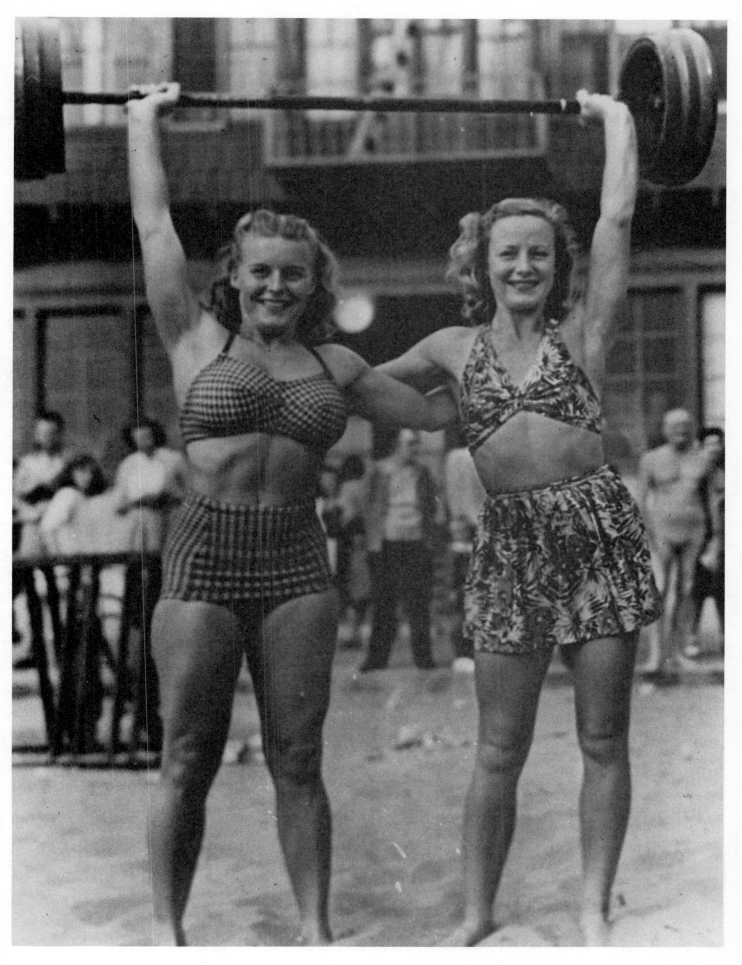

I Am the Strongest Woman Alive

I May Belong to the Weaker Sex, But--

By Marta Farra

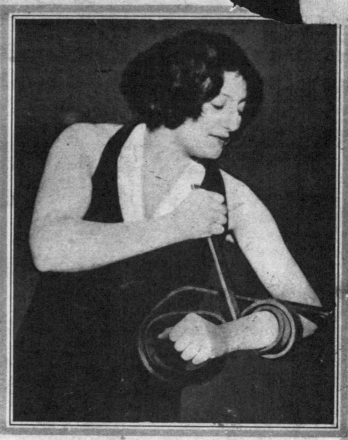

Marta Farra winding a band of steel about her arm almost as easily as though it were tape.

I AM the strongest woman in the world.

That is a broad statement, but I have demonstrated its truth hundreds of times; am doing it every day, in fact, as a part of my regular work as a professional strong woman and all-'round athlete.

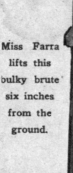

Miss Farra lifts this bulky brute six inches from the ground.

Let me cite a single circumstance that you may visualize my physical powers—particularly astonishing, especially when you consider that they are possessed by one of the so-called "weaker sex."

Louis Cyr, premier weight-lifting marvel and monarch of all strong men of recent times, lifted 4,000 pounds on his broad, bulging, muscular back, and the amazed world gasped.

Cyr weighed 375 pounds.

I can and have lifted 3,500 pounds upon my not so broad shoulders.

And I tip the scales at but 120 pounds.

The total weight I have lifted exceeds by hundreds of pounds the maximum raised by any other strong woman. Few brawny male giants have made a showing equal to mine, and some of my feats of strength never have been duplicated by any man.

Though, at first glance, I do not give the impression of being the superlatively strong woman I really am—because of my comparatively light weight and medium height—I rejoice in the fact that my achievements have caused the press and the public to confer upon me the titles of "The Feminine Hercules" and "The Atlas of the Fair Sex."

Give me a bar of cold, stubborn steel, and I will fashion it into a horseshoe with my bare hands.

Let me rest my bare back upon a plank studded with long, sharp spikes—a "torture bed" that would feaze the bravest soldier who ever dared pointed bayonets and snapping machine-guns—and I will support upon my chest 3,000 pounds of stone.

And, while I am thus weighted down, with the needle-like spikes trying to tear into my back in a thousand places, you may bring on the best sledge hammer manipulators in America and let them try to make me wince or whimper while they pound away with their mightiest swings.

And I can take a man's place in the squared circle, on the mat or in the gym, and more than hold my own. For I have as many knockouts to my credit as many men who have achieved championship honors with the mitts, and I know the wrestling game from A to Z.

But, if you have not seen me, do not picture me as an over-developed freak, with bulging muscles which rob my figure of all beauty of contour and a face lined and hard from years of training and persistent exertion.

For the contrary is the case.

I possess a face and figure of which any prima donna might be proud, and the good looks and form which God gave me have been enhanced by my mode of living.

Some women are content with a beautiful face. But there is no genuine beauty unless the body is as splendid as the features. And, as the beautiful body will remain only if carefully nurtured and systematically exercised, I insist that the athletically developed woman is bound to be more beautiful than her less energetic sisters.

How did I reach my present state of physical perfection?

I will tell you.

My mother and father were acrobats—the best in all Italy and the descendants of a long line of professional performers—and, probably because of this, I was born with a perfectly formed body and a naturally strong and robust constitution.

They did not understand physical culture, as it long has been interpreted here through the medium of magazines and books, but they followed its precepts, which had been part of the Farra family training for generations.

Fresh air aplenty, systematic exercises, work in the open and careful eating were features of the program to which none of them ever thought of making objection. It was just an accepted part of our lives—because of which we were healthy, strong and lived long—and that was all there was to it. We would no more have thought of weakening our bodies with abuses or excesses than we would have thought of defaming our native land.

For doctors we had little use, except when accidents made it necessary to have broken bones reset; and medicines almost never reached our stomachs.

Since coming to this country and reading about the splendidly organized courses in physical training in vogue here, I have been delighted to know that I have, since

babyhood, been a follower of physical culture's principles.

Perhaps it would not be too much if the exponents of modern physical culture claimed me as the outstanding example of their teachings among the women of the world.

I was born in Florence, Italy, in a very humble quarter of the city, just twenty-one years ago. The flags were flying from the government buildings and the housetops that day. However, this was not in honor of my initial appearance on the earth, but because it was a feast day. In fact, as there was nothing about the newest member of the Farra family to indicate that she would one day rank as the world's strongest woman, the advent of the nine-pound, black-eyed infant attracted no attention outside of our immediate circle.

I was, then, just a normal baby, just an addition to the Farras, destined to be reared carefully and trained thoroughly to become a professional acrobat. And the training began almost as soon as I could toddle, though I still recollect that, in my early years, I had a feeling that might, strength and brawn should be masculine qualities, and that I would have been better pleased to have been permitted to grow up dainty and allowed more time to play with my dolls and wear pretty clothes.

Nothing indicative of the feminine Hercules to be in that, was there? In fact, had I been given my choice then between becoming the world's strongest woman and a replica of Dante's Beatrice, I know I should have chosen to be the latter.

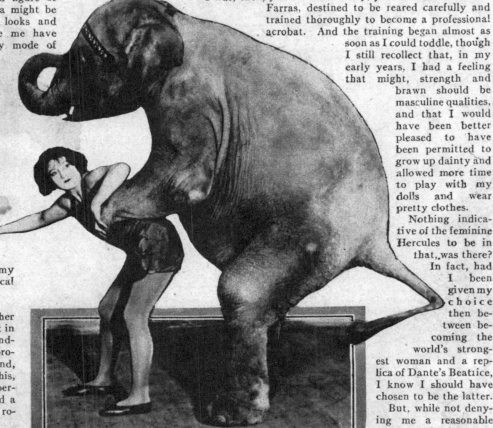

They are not playing leap frog. Miss Farra and her elephant are posing to show the disparity in their sizes. The little one can lift the big one.

But, while not denying me a reasonable amount of play, my parents put me through a long and sometimes tedious course of training to prepare me for the acrobatic career to come. When but eleven years of age, I made my first appearance behind the footlights as one of the team of which my father and mother were the stars, and by the time I was twelve, looked upon the rings as almost my constant companions.

And not only did I come to like the work, but I lived true to the ethics of our profession, learning every trick of the trade that I might carry on when my parents retired and take the fame of the Farra acrobats into another generation.

Then came my first engagement with a circus, a change ever to be remembered. To be able to travel with a circus long has been the great ambition of every red-blooded boy and girl, and I was no exception. When my mother told me the great news, that they were quitting the stage to perform under canvas, I was the happiest girl in all Italy. I could hardly wait for the signing (Continued on page 42)

"I've got everything going for me—balance, symmetry, and I'm very female-looking; I don't look extremely masculine, whatever masculine is."
—Rachel McLish

competition and then from women's bodybuilding altogether.

Lisa Lyon was quoted in 1981 as saying, "I started this sport. It's not my fault other women want to take it further."

Despite her contributions to it, Lisa Lyon did not start the sport, as we have seen—any more or less than Joan of Arc did. She was not even very much in evidence at its birth. But she was right about this: by 1981 there were other women, quite a few of them, who were willing to take it further, now that it was hatched and—largely because of Lisa and Doris Barrilleaux—organized and sanctioned and even televised. By then there were women who were willing to take it as far as it would go.

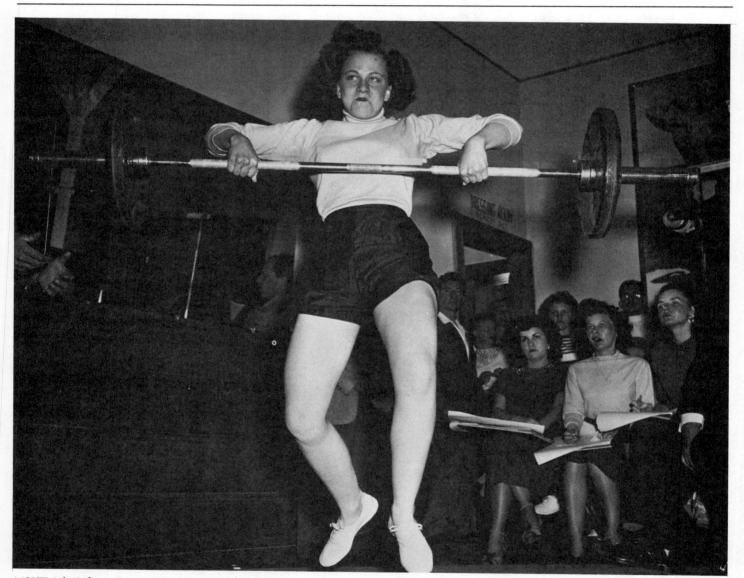

AAU Weight-Lifting Competition, Los Angeles, 1950

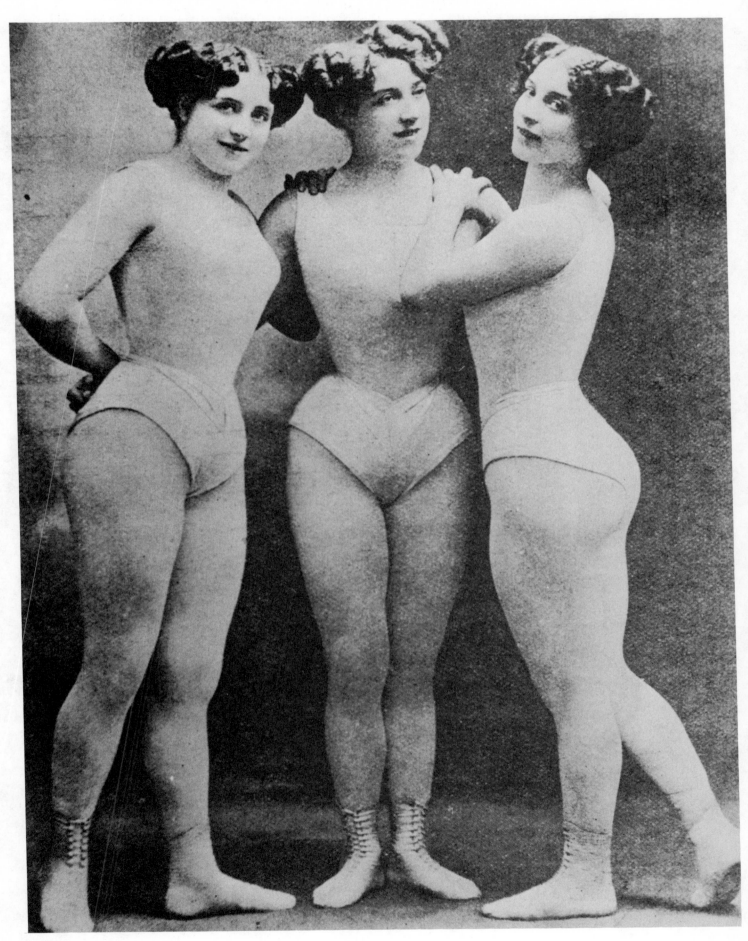

Amazon Triplets, 19th century

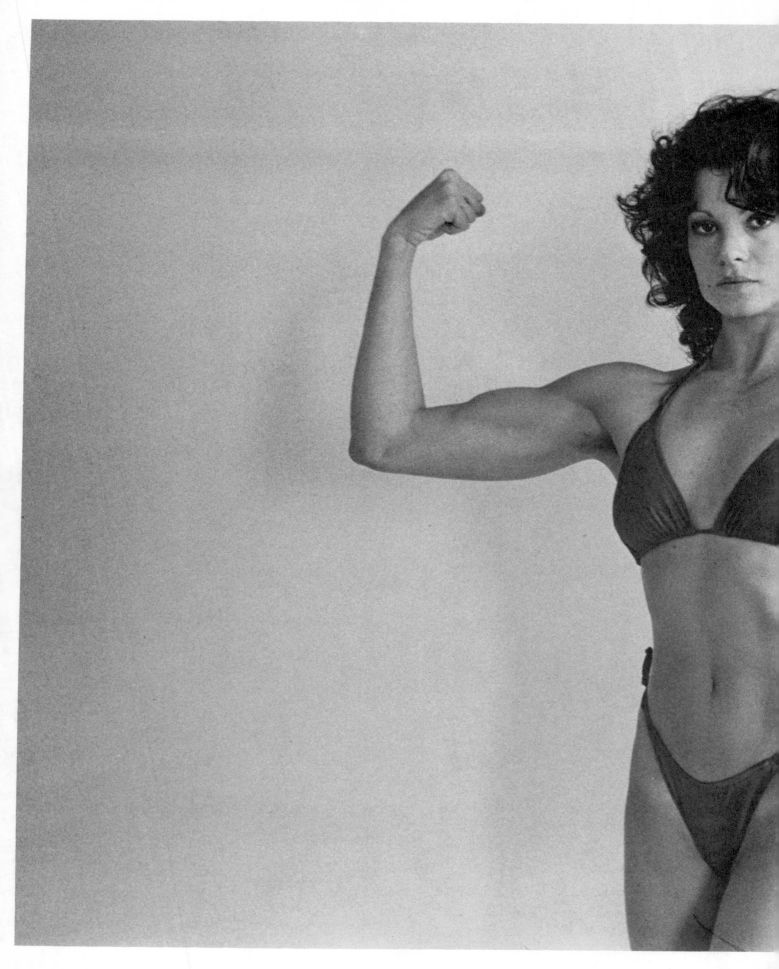

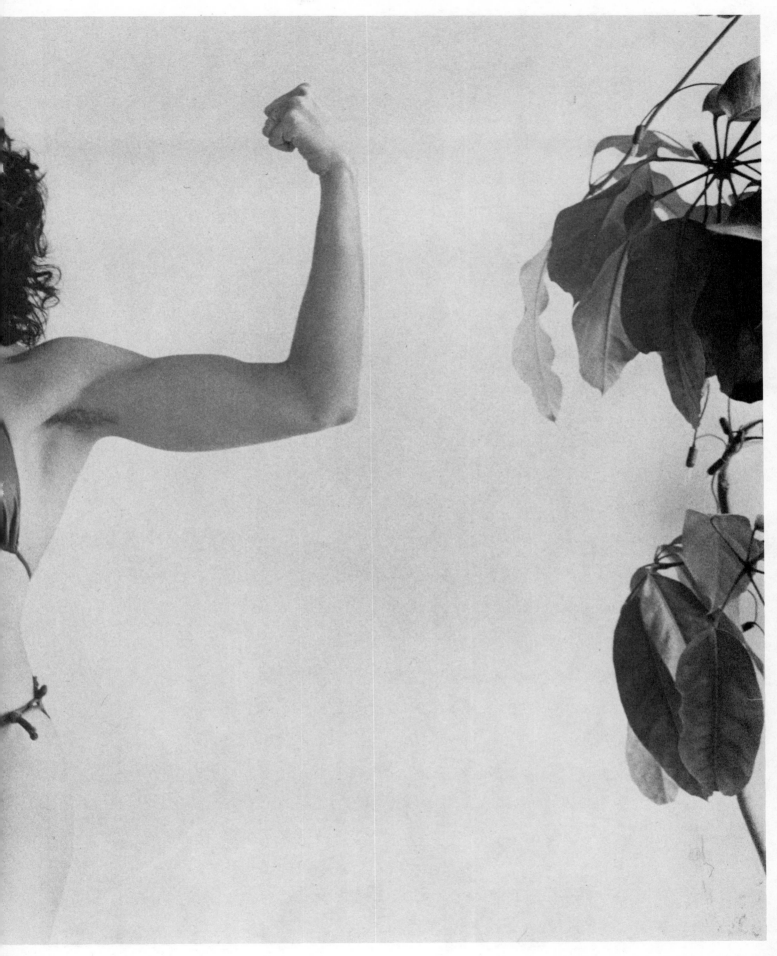

Lisa Lyon

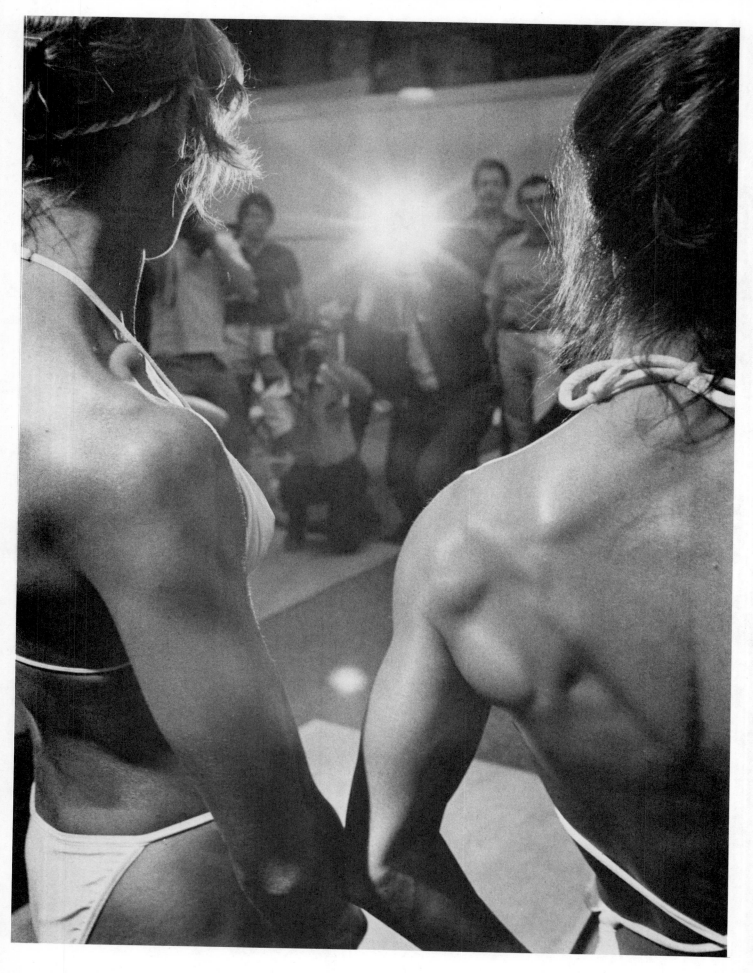

3

Television took to women's bodybuilding like lint to wool, and before it was really even here. The program called *Real People* filmed a segment on a contest in Tampa as early as 1979. In 1980 NBC's *Sports World* covered the U.S. Women's Bodybuilding Championship in Atlantic City, which was won by Rachel McLish shortly before she won the first Miss Olympia contest the same year. And in 1981, after the sport was really and truly born, after there were organizations and guidelines and after Lisa Lyon had retired, NBC covered that contest again. Its name was changed to the World Women's Bodybuilding Championship; it was opened to both professionals and a few amateurs, included a couples' competition (a man and a woman posing together); and it was second in total prize money and prestige only to the Miss Olympia. And by the time that contest was held, less than a year after the sport had arrived, television had women's bodybuilding all figured out—it had recognized the profound, irreconcilable aesthetic division at the heart of it and had determined how to exploit it.

As Lisa Lyon had foreseen there would be, as there had to be, there were two camps by then. There were the women on whom muscles showed only when they flexed, women who wanted and achieved through the use of weights bodies which were at best only slightly more muscular than female gymnasts' and dancers', and whose key aesthetic concerns were femininity and symmetry. And then there were the others, the "freaks" as some people called them, the group that had burgeoned around Auby Paulick and Cammie Lusko from that first Miss Olympia contest to include by 1981 five or six other top competitive representatives. These women wanted nothing to do with beauty-contest aesthetics. They wanted *muscles,* and they were interested not only in taking women's bodybuilding further, as Lisa Lyon claimed they had, but, in the words of a popular song of that year, to "Take It to the Limit"—to the max.

It was clear to television that viewers would be cu-rious about this second group of women. That people would tune in in droves to see women with muscles like men, even if many of those people were offended by it. It was also clear to NBC that many of their viewers *would* be offended by it. The network's unofficial position, therefore (reportedly, this position was actually *stated* to one of the producers of the '81 World Women's Bodybuilding Championship), seemed to go something like this: We want to *see* a lot of these freaky, muscular types, but we *definitely* don't want one of them to win.

It's an ambivalent position for an ambivalent situation, one which television, certainly, had nothing to do with creating; but the position has filtered down through television to the public and it now poses the central and biggest dilemma of women's bodybuilding: if it is to make it as a spectator sport, if it is to transcend its lack of historical archetype and *make it,* as anything bigger than, say, midget wrestling, as competition before a paying public, then what exactly *is* that competition? What should win women's bodybuilding contests, and what should not? And why?

There were four particularly muscular women at the '81 World Women's Bodybuilding Championship. One of them, Lisa Elliott, who was more muscular than any woman there, was given a lot of air time by NBC but did not place; another, Laura Combes, the amateur champion of 1980, placed sixth. The winner of the competition, and co-winner with Chris Dickerson of the couples' competition, was a tiny, dainty, pert-faced gymnast named Lynn Conkwright, who weighs one hundred three pounds and doesn't have a single big muscle to her name.

"Quality muscle is what I want. That, and proportion," says Lynn Conkwright. She is training with Rachel McLish and twelve or fourteen other women at a brand-new gym called the Olympus in Bristol, Pennsylvania. It is a Thursday, August 20, two days before the 1981 Miss Olympia Contest which will be held

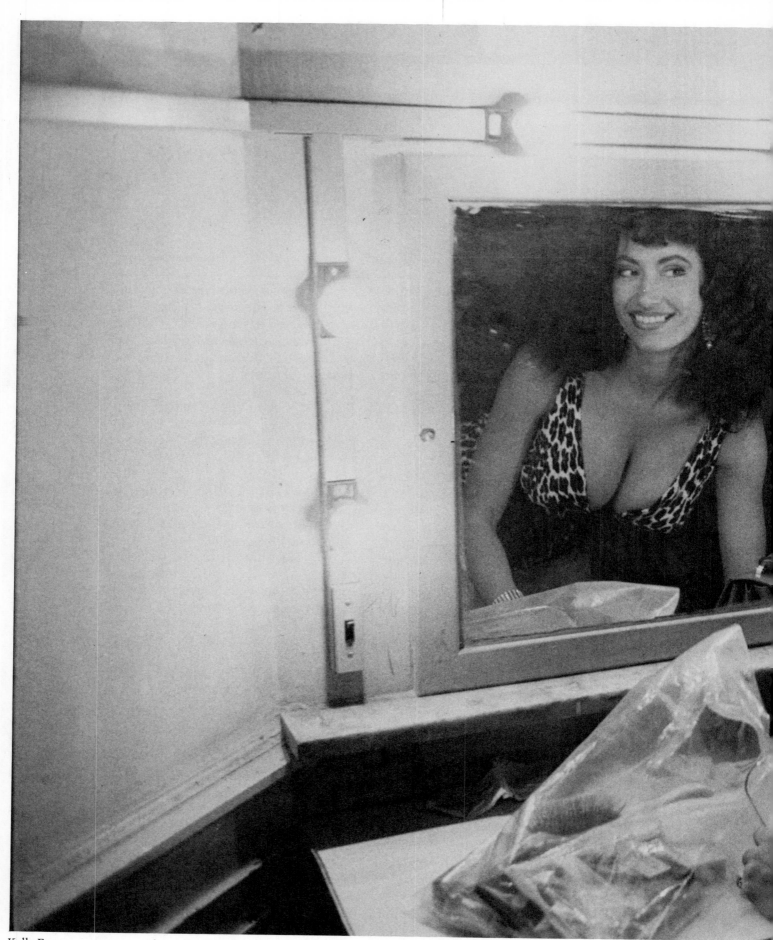

Kelly Everts, contestant, early women's bodybuilding competition. Brooklyn Academy of Music, 1973

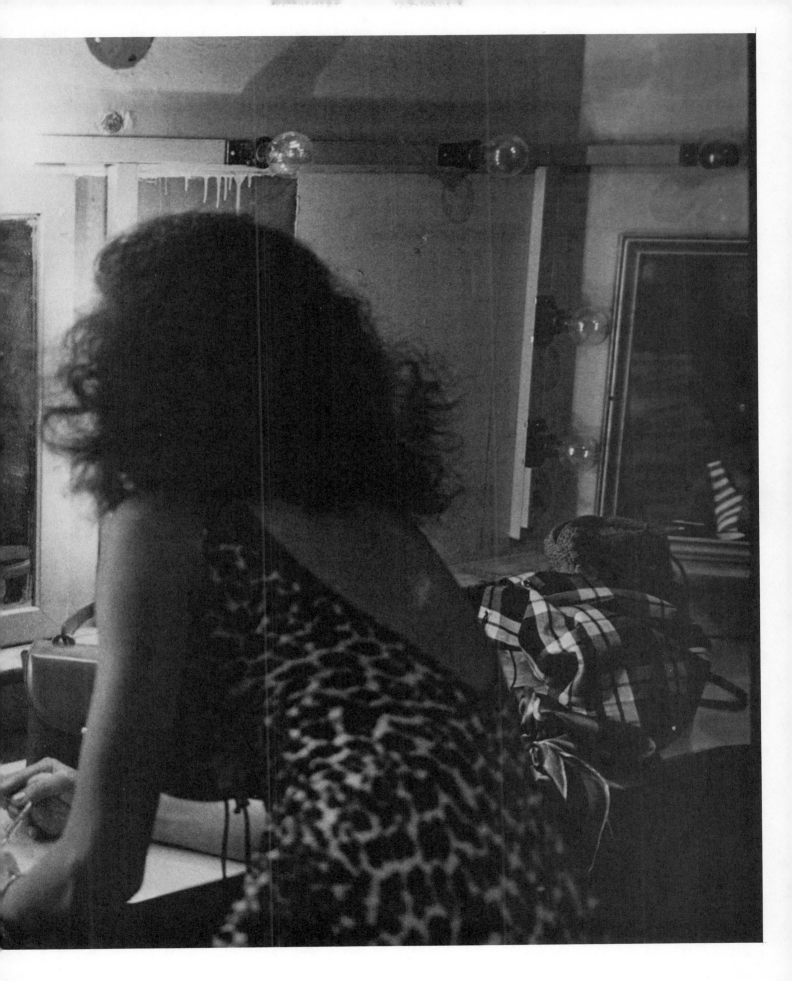

again at the Sheraton Hotel in Philadelphia, and George Snyder, the contest promoter, has brought these women out here thirty miles from Philadelphia to get in one last workout before the competition and to celebrate the gym's opening day. The gym is a big, airy, warehouselike place with tall windows looking out onto a highway. It is full of Snyder-built equipment and decorated with outsized posters of Arnold and Franco and other male bodybuilding stars, though the owners claim the gym is geared to serve women.

There are a lot of people in the workout area watching the women train, among them Ricky Wayne, the bodybuilding writer, and members of a video crew from Delaware County, here making a film of the competition for Snyder, who hopes to sell it to cable tele-

vision. The women ignore the camera, as they have learned to do recently, and answer questions between sets of exercises—questions mostly directly to the central divisive issue in their sport, the big-muscles-versus-femininity issue. That issue is on a lot of minds here today because Laura Combes, whom some people believe to be the best of the big-muscle competitors, is entered in this year's Miss Olympia, and is said to be in much better shape than she was in when Lynn Conkwright beat her a couple of months ago. Nobody knows, as usual, precisely what the judges will be looking for. Lynn Conkwright has stayed in exactly the same shape that won her the World Women's Championship; Rachel McLish is ten pounds heavier than she was for last year's Miss Olympia, at which, she feels, she

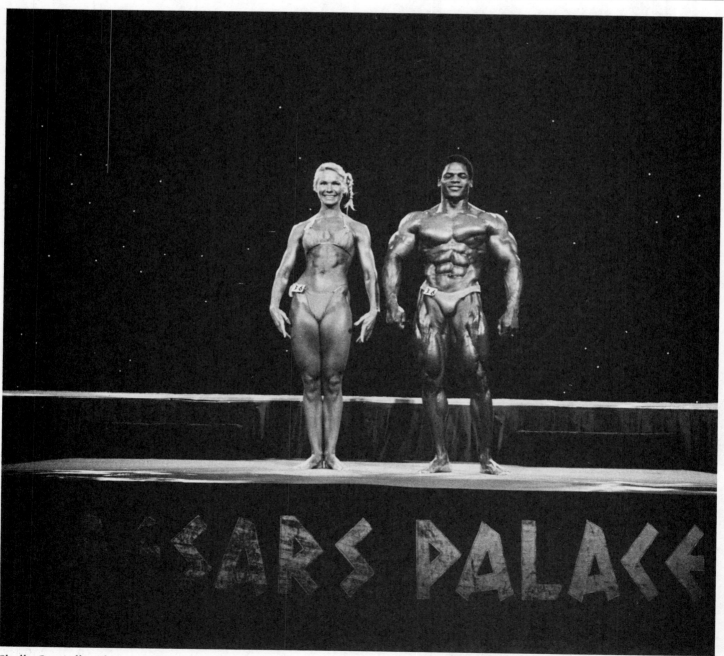

Shelly Gruwell and Tony Pierson, Las Vegas

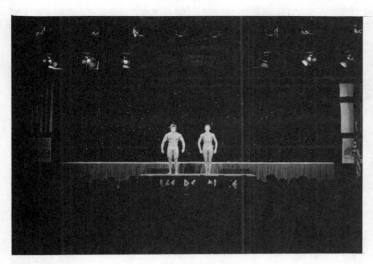

"I really don't enjoy posing that much. I'd rather give a bodybuilding seminar instead of doing a guest-posing appearance, because I really don't enjoy getting up there in a little bitty skimpy bikini and strutting my stuff. For competition I will, because it's required and I want to do my best. I do enjoy it for competition, but not just for show at all."
—Rachel McLish

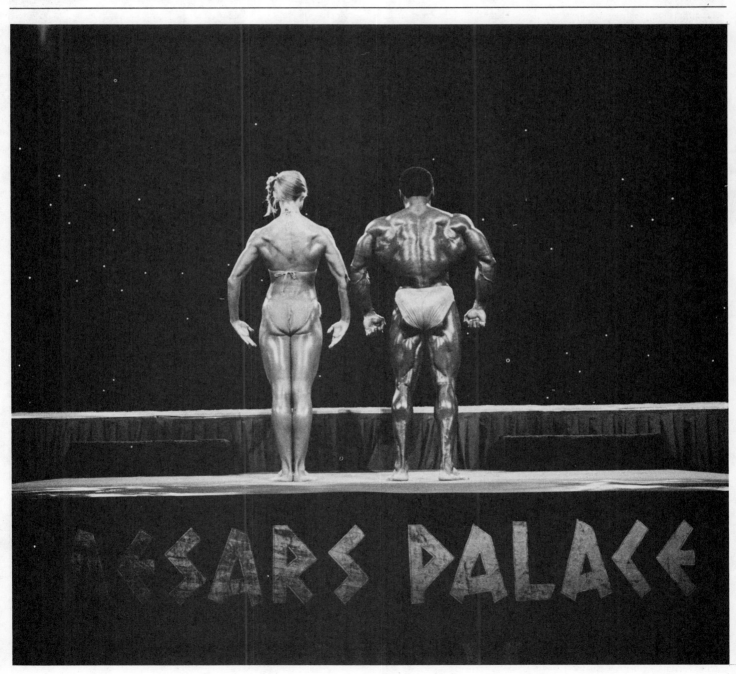

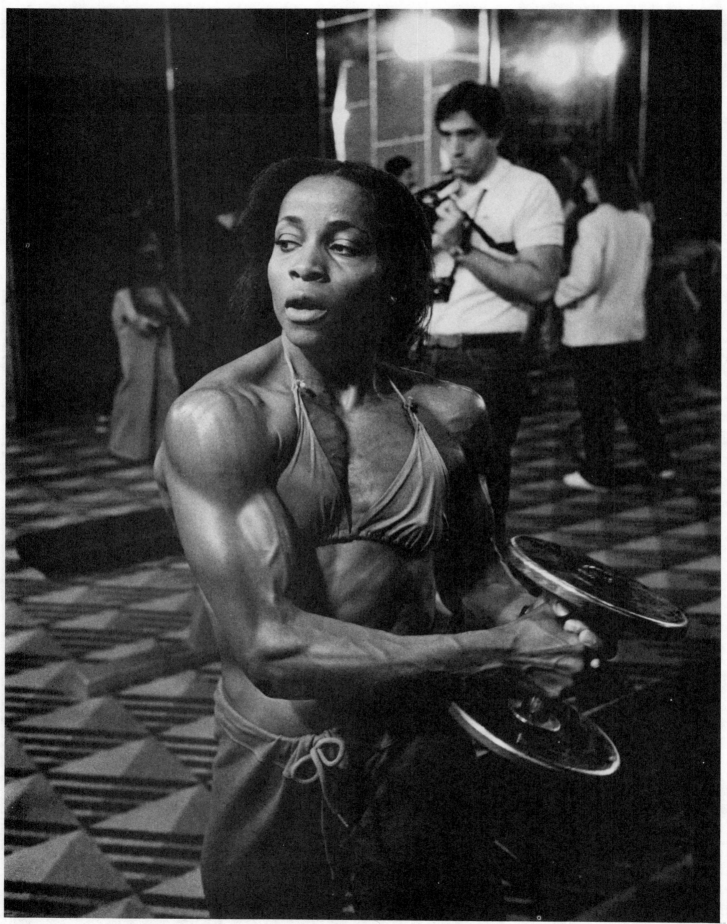

Carla Dunlap, Atlantic City, 1981

looked too cut-up and scrawny.

"I just want to look like a fit, healthy, good-looking woman," says Rachel, regarding herself in one of the big wall mirrors.

"Don't worry, darlin'," says Ellen Davis, who is doing stomach twists on a bench behind Rachel. "You do." Ellen Davis calls everybody "darlin'." She is a pretty, ironic, blowsy woman of thirty-two, the wife of body-builder Steve Davis, who is here training with her. She is dressed in a black leotard, mauve tights and white Peugeot cycling gloves to protect her hands from calluses.

"Until I flex," adds Rachel. She flexes her right biceps at the mirror and a thin muscle jumps to attention. "Then people can see." Rachel is wearing an elegant pair of black knit tights, a gold belt and a gold and turquoise star necklace. Her dark, glossy hair is in a jaunty ponytail and everything about her, from her grave, lovely, Byzantine face to her fingers and wrists and small feet, has a unifying sheen to it. The ten pounds have filled her out, particularly in the chest and buttocks; if she is less defined than she was last year, she is certainly healthier looking, and health is the word that keeps cropping up here among these women, not one of whom is a big-muscle type.

"There are so many misconceptions about women's bodybuilding. What we're really going for is fit, shapely, healthy bodies, and for general overall health," says Rachel McLish.

Lynn Conkwright gets up from a bench where she

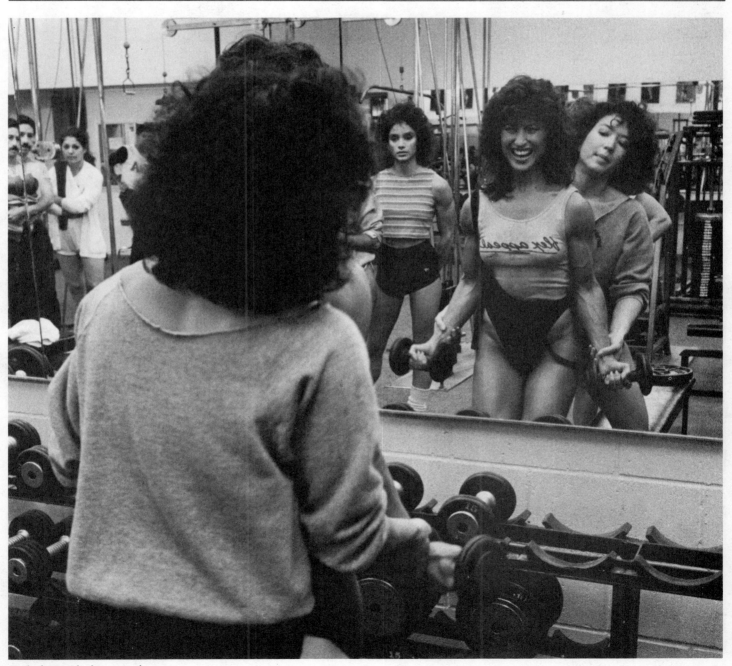

Rachel McLish doing curls

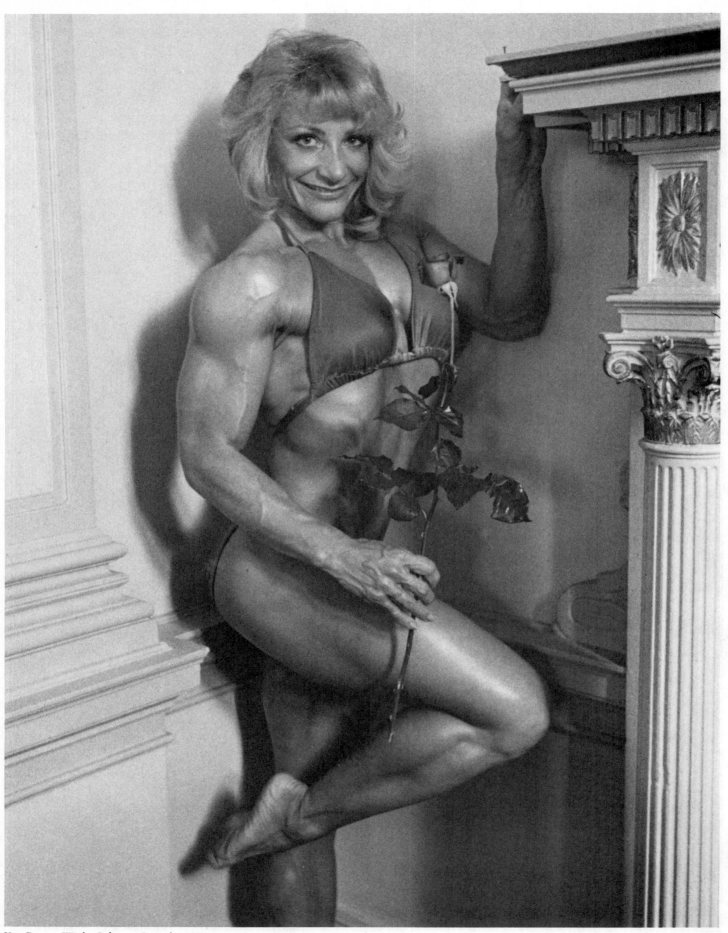

Kay Baxter-Wick, Calgary, Canada, 1983

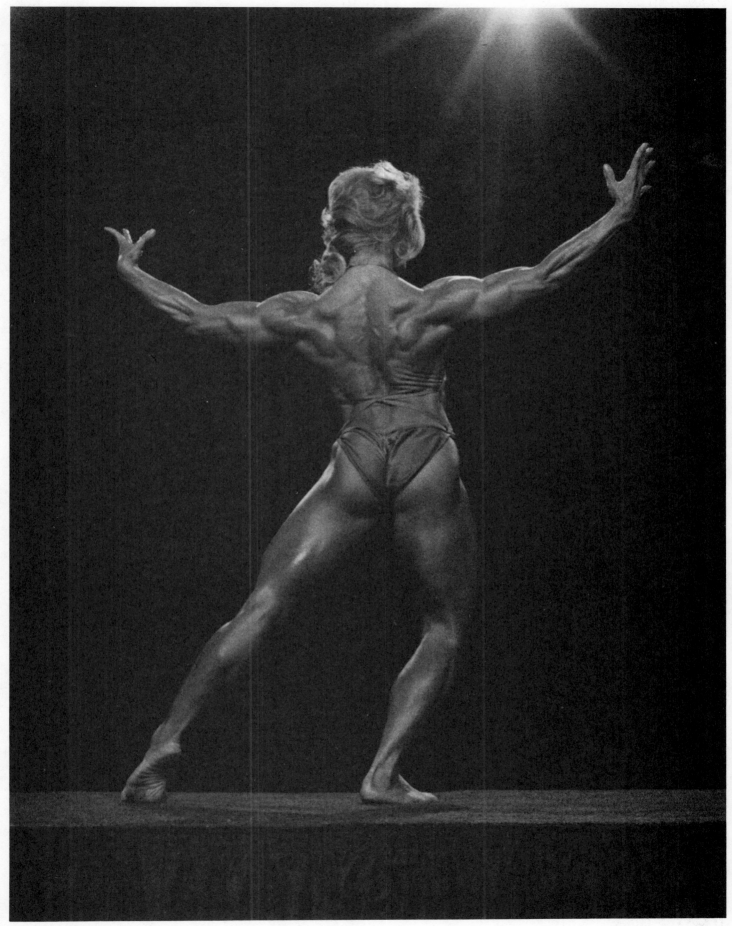

Kay Baxter-Wick

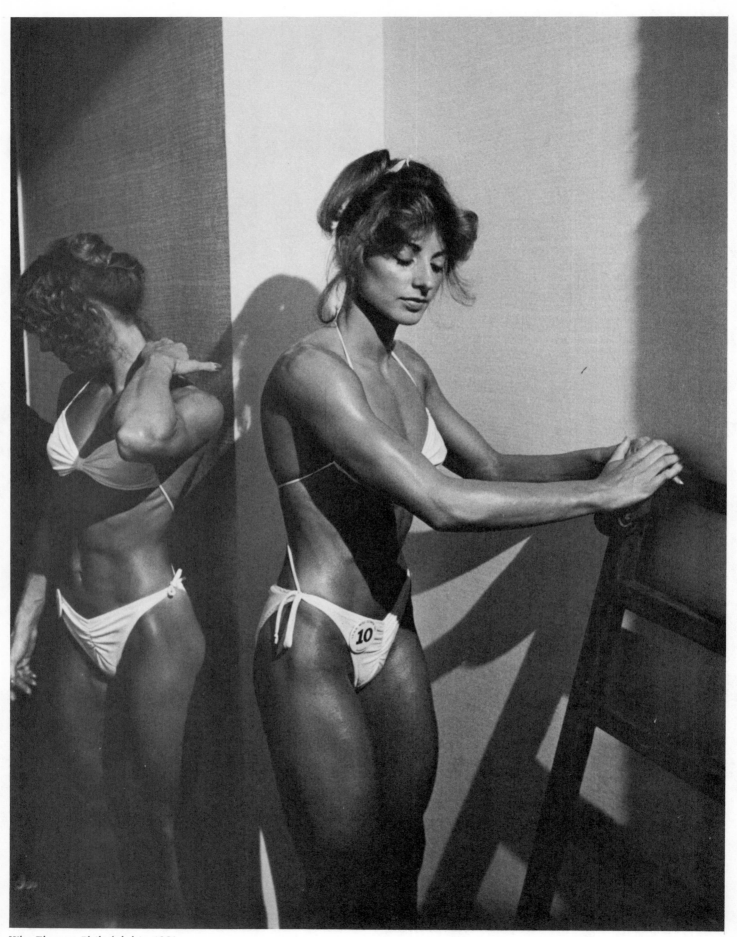

Kike Elomaa, Philadelphia, 1981

has been doing narrow-grip bench presses with sixty pounds on a bar.

"Muscles have their place—on stage," she says. "But never too many. Some women carry it too far, *do* want to be men. We don't. We want to be *women*—we want the muscularity to enhance our femininity. I can honestly say I've done everything with my body I want to up to this point. It pleases me to know that women all over the world now want to look *better*—they want to be firm and look good, and that's bodybuilding too."

"Then why compete?" someone asks her.

"To get the word out to other women," Lynn and Rachel say at the same time. "To spread the word."

"I've never enjoyed the stage performance part of competition," says Rachel. "I hate it. I'm not an exhibitionist."

"I don't know," says Lynn. "For me, performing is my way of showing the audience that muscles can look good on a woman."

What muscles she has look very good indeed on Lynn Conkwright. At five feet and one hundred three pounds, she has a taut, dainty, athlete's body, with beautifully developed legs and a symmetrical torso. She also has a sincere, generous face, a country-sunshine smile, wide blue eyes, a sweet, demure personality and a quick mind. If you were to wonder what sort of women become female bodybuilders, you couldn't find a more prototypical example than Lynn Conkwright, who is so representative of her sisters in the sport that the cloth might have been cut directly

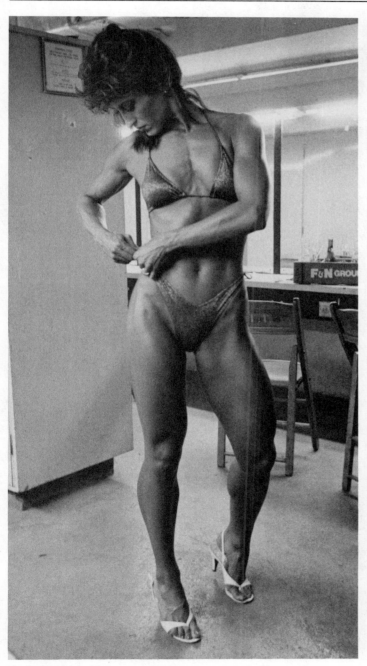

Rachel McLish, Singapore, 1983

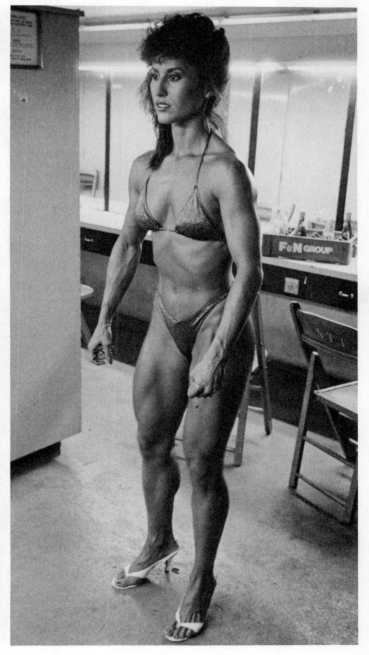

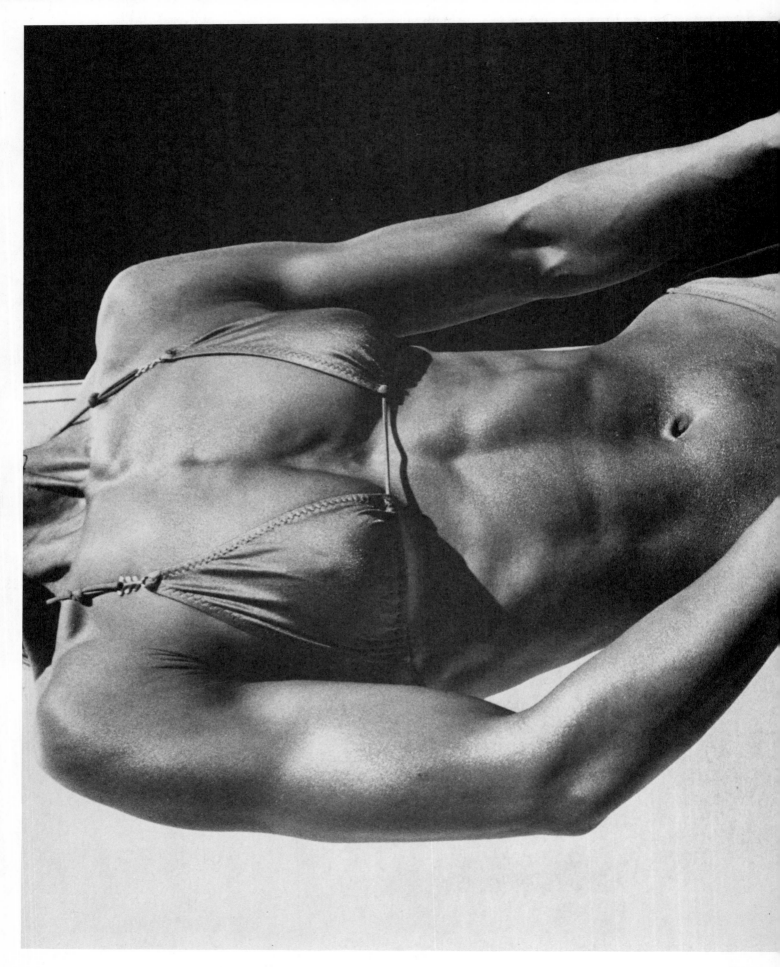

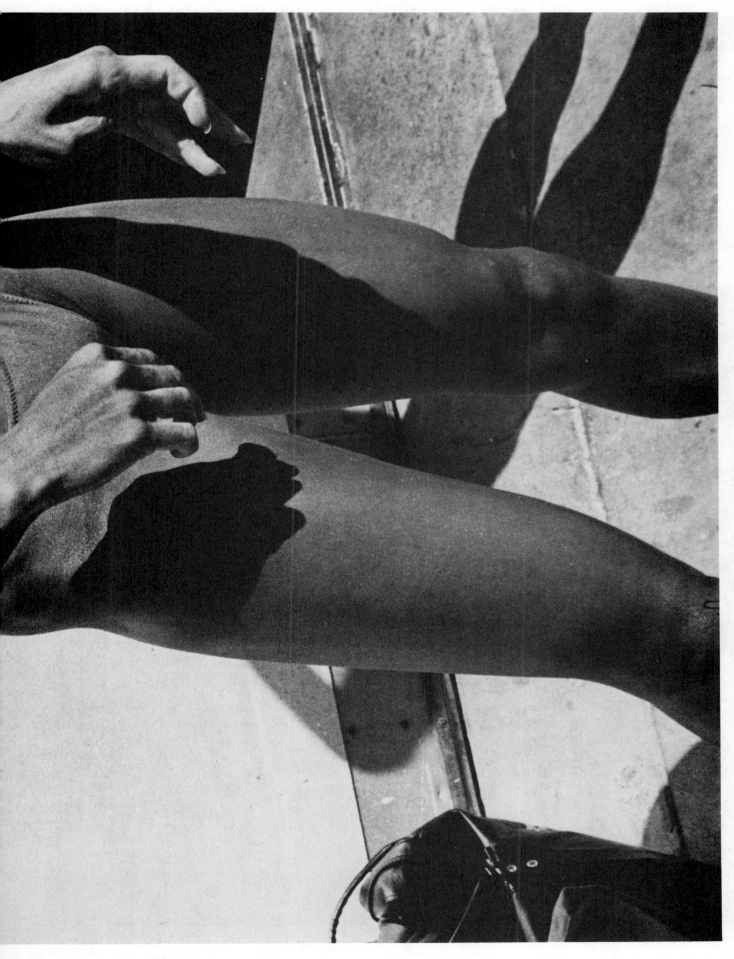

from her. Like most of the others, she is in her middle twenties and comes from a middle-class background which afforded her a college education, conventional middle-America values and an early introduction to sports. Typically also, she is happily married, lives in a nonurban environment, is bright and cheerful, and has been athletic for most of her life. It was to get stronger for competitive gymnastics that Lynn took up using weights in college, and she still coaches gymnastics and track at a high school in Virginia Beach, Virginia, near the farm on which she and her husband live. She also skis, and surfs well enough to have taken a sixth place in an East Coast surfing championship.

What Lynn Conkwright is not also goes for most other female bodybuilders: she is not urban or very sophisticated, she is not at all dumb or dikey, revolutionary, oversexed, or illiterate. She is not blue-collar or a drug user or a boozer or a feminist or a groupie. Rather, she is a pretty, pert, slightly tomboyish All-American Girl who grew up eating peanut-butter-and-jelly sandwiches and going to slumber parties, a Betty out of the *Archie* comic books, a member of the "nice girl" sorority who always had good grades and played on the field hockey team. What made her different from other girls of her age and background was that her own body was her best friend; from early on its health and good looks were the source of her biggest pleasures, and so she made it her way of life.

The women talk sweetly to each other as they train, hugging and giggling sometimes like little girls, and

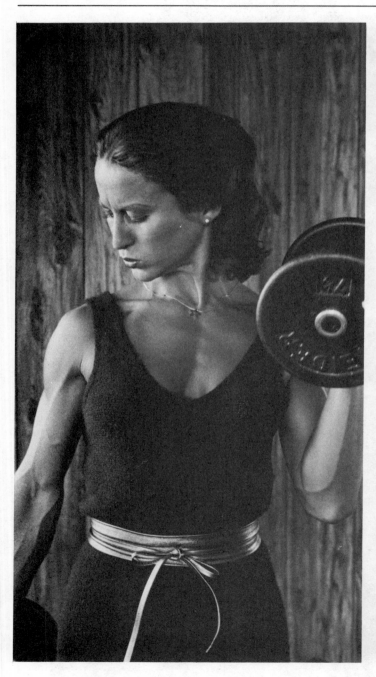
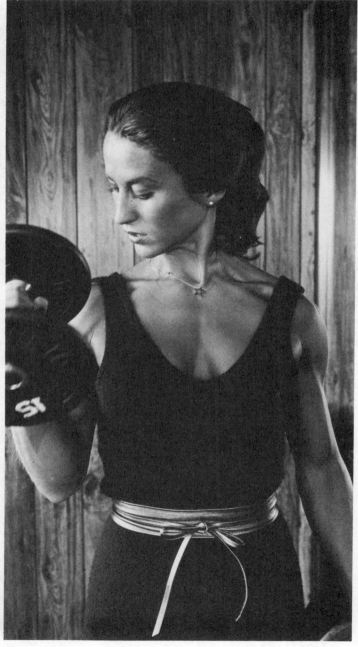

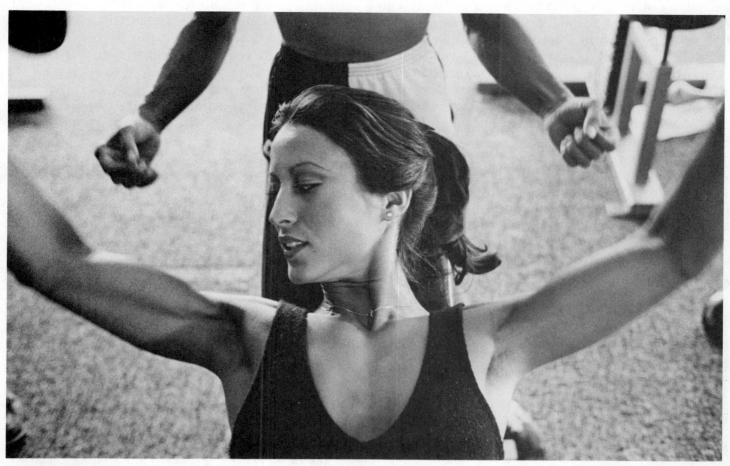

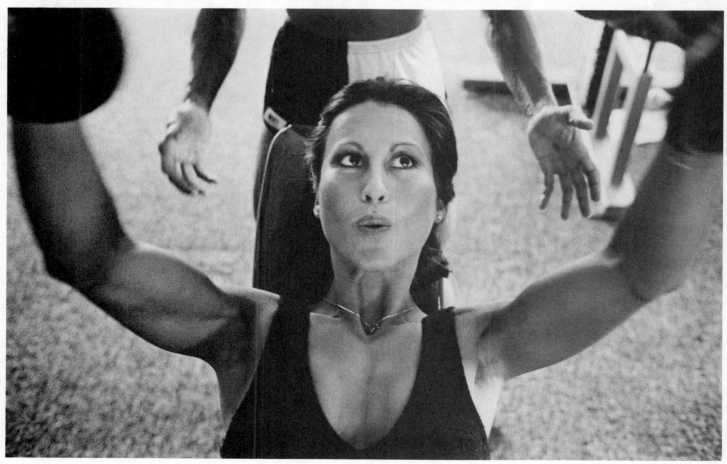

talking about flyes, dips, cuts. They are not as self-conscious as male bodybuilders, and there is less symbolic pouting and grimacing when they pose in front of the mirrors. They look at their tanned, well-shaped bodies the way women have always regarded themselves in mirrors, with unemotional, appraising eyes, and they giggle and touch and enjoy each other like girls at a sorority party, and talk about the thing they do with their lives.

In the past year Rachel McLish has been to Venezuela, Japan, Scandinavia, Canada and England promoting women's bodybuilding. Lynn Conkwright has been to Taiwan and Venezuela, and has trips planned to South Africa, Bali, and the Philippines. Spreading the word.

"This sport is just starting," says Lynn.

"And I'm telling you," adds Rachel, "all over the *world*."

"Do you see yourselves getting rich and famous from it?" I asked them.

"No," says Lynn.

"Yes," says Rachel definitively.

"Well," adds Lynn. She thinks, then grins. "Maybe later."

The talk turns to steroids, the synthetic male hormone drugs widely used by male bodybuilders and strength athletes, and now said to be used by some female bodybuilders. All the women here claim never to have used drugs and to loathe the idea of doing so. Rachel McLish irritably bounces her ponytail at the

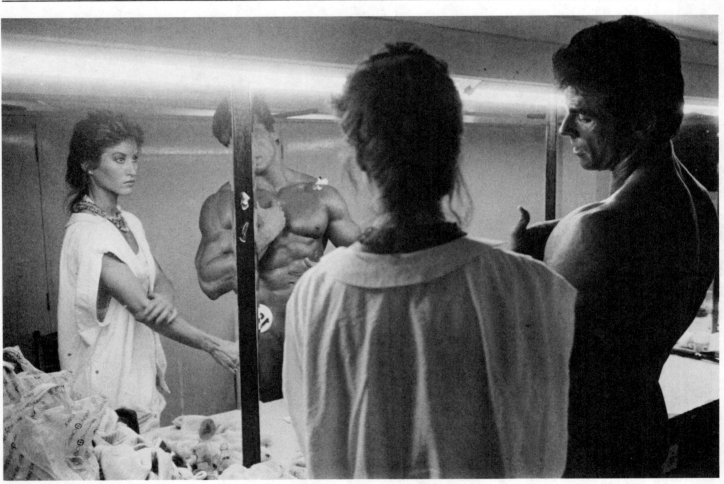

Rachel in Singapore

subject and says, much as Archie's Betty might, "I don't think women who use steroids will ever win national contests. What wins is hard training, good nutrition, emotional stability and good mental attitude."

Aside from Rachel and Lynn and April Nicotra—a curvy, smart brunette who was twice a winner of the old Miss Americana contest and others of the premuscle, high-heeled, bathing-beauty-type competitions—none of the women here knows much about winning national contests. For Candy Csencsits, for instance, a cheerful, very pretty twenty-five-year-old gymnast and former phys-ed teacher from Allentown, Pennsylvania, this is her first big competition—and she is happy to be here. Candy wears a red leotard, red and white shorts, has a lot of brown hair tousled on top of her head, a constant, infectious grin, and sports a diamond-studded twenty-four-carat tiny barbell on a gold chain around her neck. Her biggest ambition is to win the Miss Olympia contest. Asked if she thinks she will do that, she says, "Well . . . yes. A lot of judges tell me my back is the best they've seen—that there aren't many girls with a perfect diamond like mine."

Donna Frame likes her back too, and believes that she also has a chance of winning the contest. Donna is from Fremont, California, is Miss Western USA and a former Oakland Raider cheerleader. She is tall and very feminine, with gray hair and a sensitive face. She wants to win the Olympia and then go on and win the couples competition in Atlantic City with Arnold Schwarzenegger as her partner. Does she know Ar-

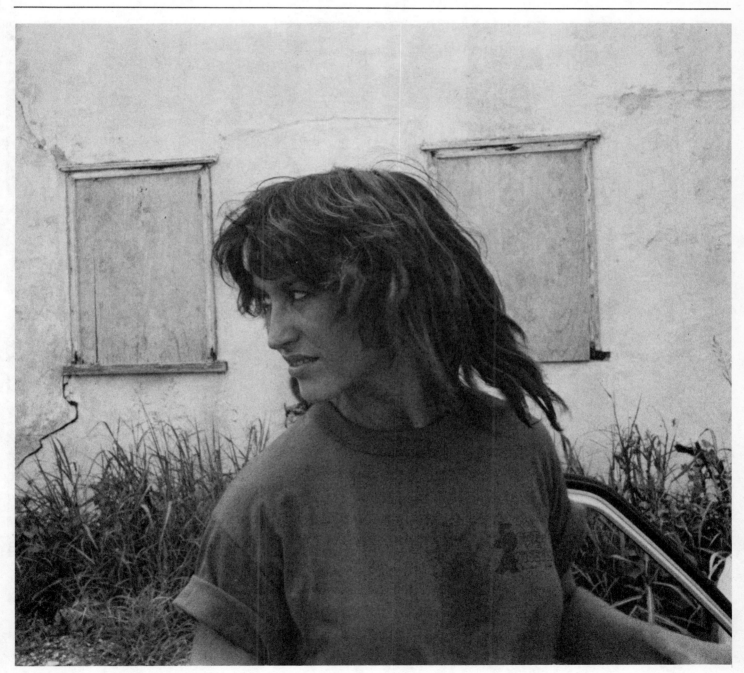

Rachel at home in Harlingen, Texas

nold? she is asked. No . . . but she plans to meet him.

The training begins to tail off. Lynn Conkwright describes having her legs waxed to a group of the women. She and Rachel pose together for George Butler, and after the picture a tall black man who has been watching the workout all afternoon walks over and, following a polite request, begins feeling different parts of Rachel, testing them experimentally with his fingers as if they were melons.

Murray, a short, freckled, heavy-chested gym instructor at the Olympus, watches the feeling going on with his chunky arms crossed, grinning. Ricky Wayne asks him if muscular women turn him on. "I might be a little attracted to it," says Murray. "In an aspect they do. Some of them do and some don't. There's one brute

that turns me on. Smooth ones turn me on some too."

"Do you think a woman looks good ripped?" asked Wayne, who is prodding now and amused.

"I'm not turned on by a woman who is ripped . . . but I'm not turned off either. I *really* like tall, thin women . . ." Murray looks up at Ricky Wayne. "How about you, woman bodybuilders turn you on?"

"Rachel does," says Wayne. "I think she has a perfect body. But male bodybuilding has had too much to say about all this. Women ought to be allowed to make their own aesthetic decisions. If they were, there wouldn't be all this confusion about standards. It's men like Mike Mentzer [a top male bodybuilder] who have told these woman they ought to look like men. The women want money, TV, media stuff—so they go

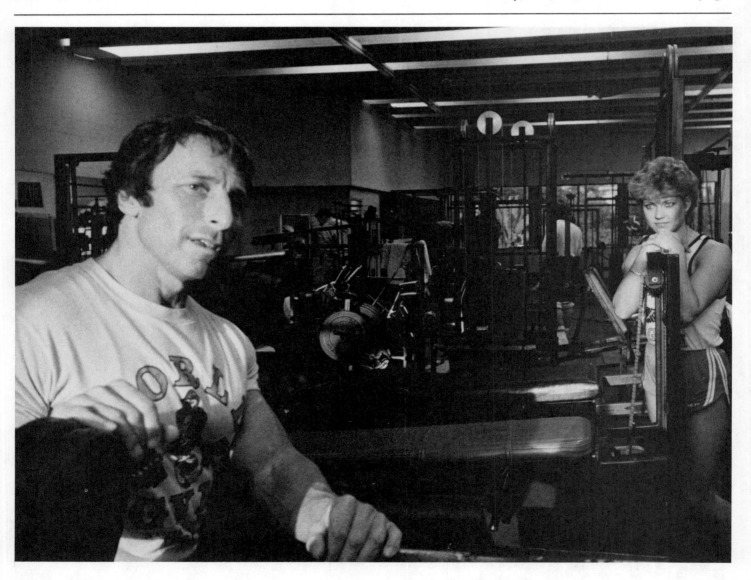

along."

The act of getting their bodies into shape, Wayne goes on to say, is great. It is competition that throws everything off. "Then they say 'Well, my thigh's well shaped, but is it *bigger* than hers?'"

On the bus back to Philadelphia, Steve Davis comments on Lynn Conkwright's perfume. "You know, I've been wearing this perfume since high school," she says. "Shalimar. And it only comes out when I sweat. It's perfect for me, isn't it? It's *perfect*."

There is more talk about foreign places to which their good bodies have taken them. Davis and his wife, Ellen, talk about skiing at Zurs and Lech. "I went all over up there," says Lynn Conkwright delightedly, making a big circle with her arm. "All over in that area."

A tall blonde tells about how when she and a girlfriend were in Paris a little bitty guy followed them into this "underthing," and so they beat him up.

"You *what*?" someone asks her.

"We beat him up. He followed us, you know, under the road into this underthing and we beat him up. Not bad, though—he ran away."

Stories are going around in the front of the bus about swimming being good for back and shoulder development, about surfing for the thighs and, as always, about diet.

"I think cantaloupe is one of the best things to eat for cuts," says Steve Davis, who, perhaps because he is married to one of them, is one of the few male body-

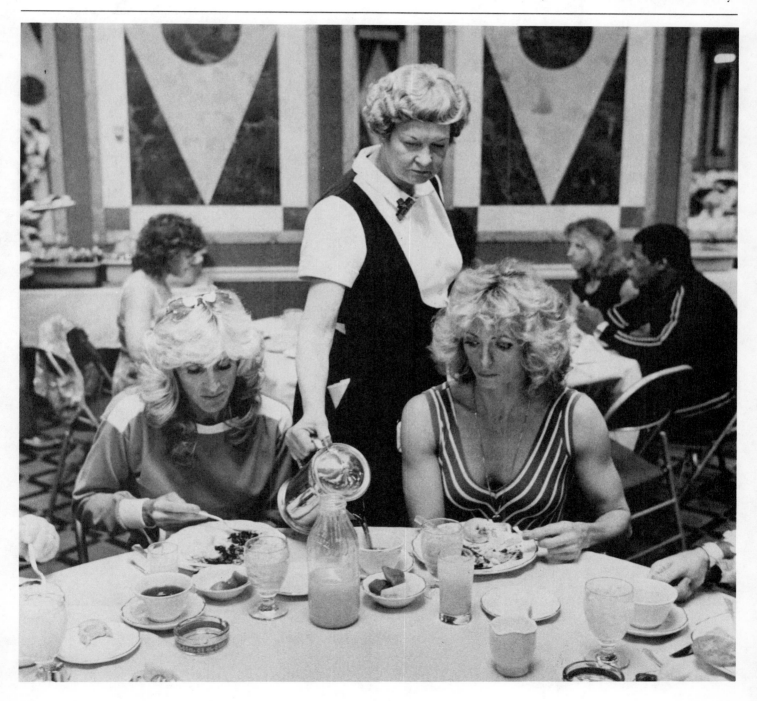

builders who seems completely at ease with these women. Many if not most male bodybuilders, including a number of the top ones, are not favorably impressed with the female version of their sport. Oddly perhaps, on the whole—and despite what they might say for the record—they tend to be more disapproving of women building muscles than is your average man on the street.

"What do you think of grapes?" Davis asks Rachel McLish.

Rachel likes grapes, it turns out, as well as cantaloupe and most other fruit. Like practically every other competitive female bodybuilder, she follows a low-fat, low-salt, low-sugar diet with little or no red meat in it, and with carefully balanced amounts of protein and carbohydrates. What this means is that female bodybuilders eat very carefully, and for good reason. Due to the male hormone, androgen, men are on the whole at least thirty percent stronger than women from late adolescence onward. They build larger muscles more quickly, and they have a higher percentage of lean body mass to fat. An average woman is twenty to twenty-five percent fat, while men average less than fifteen percent. Fat is the enemy of any bodybuilder, large or small, male or female, and because it is more of an effort for women to keep it off than for men, they tend not only to limit themselves to the traditional fruits and vegetables, chicken and fish, of all bodybuilding diets, but to eat far less of those things than their male counterparts, and to take fewer supple-

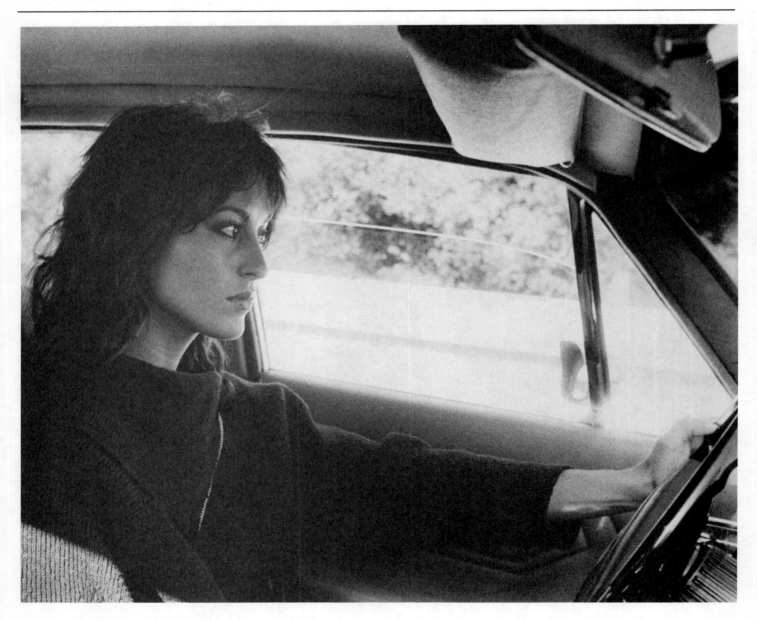

ments, in order to keep themselves at the five to ten percent body fat level deemed appropriate for their competitions. Lynn Conkwright's favorite meal, for example, is a vegetable shishkabob.

There is something magical, even sacramental, about the way male bodybuilders render the huge amounts of carefully selected food they eat into huge muscles. Turning very small amounts of food into small muscles is something else again. I have seen Ken Waller, the ex–Mr. Universe, eat at one of *three* meals on a night after competition more than all the women on this bus will eat tonight collectively. And as the conversation hovers over food, the mood going into Philadelphia, among these pleasant, pretty, athletic women, some forty hours before the biggest event of their year, grows somber for the first time all afternoon with the reminder of how little sustenance is too much for them.

Arnold Schwarzenegger was in Philadelphia that weekend, both for the contest and to be chauffeured around town in a limousine for promotion of his new book. At dinner that night, over a limitless French meal at a restaurant called The Garden, he said that he really didn't think too much of women's bodybuilding, that despite what people might think, he didn't particularly like to see women sweat.

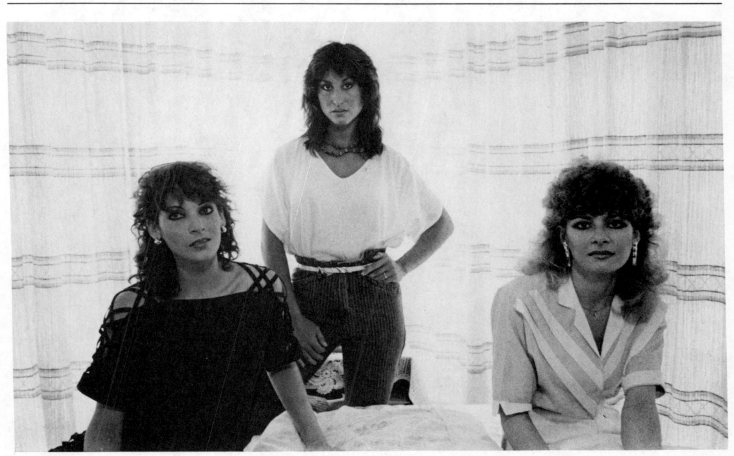

Rachel in Harlingen, Texas

71

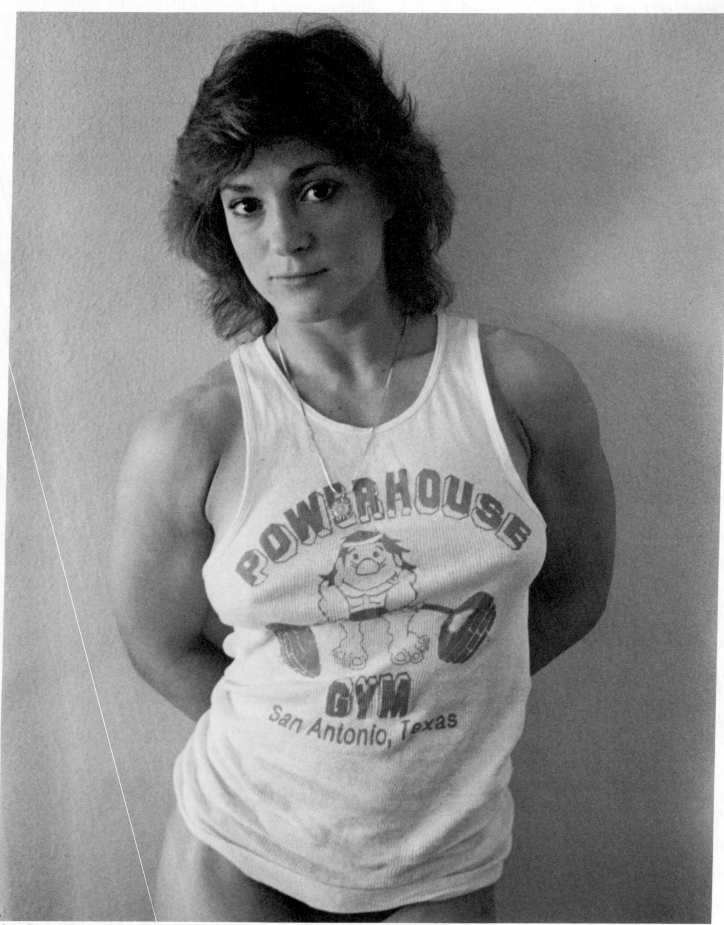

Lori Bowen, San Antonio, Texas, 1983

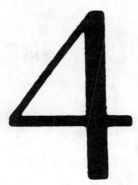

There was a lot going on in the Philadelphia Sheraton Hotel on the day before the 1981 Miss Olympia contest. In the lobby where contestants were checking in, some of them surrounded by friends and fans, most of them dressed in tight shorts, their lovely legs winking at the tourists, the place had the feel of a real, if exotic, sporting event. There were writers and photographers there doing books on women's bodybuilding, and *Mademoiselle* magazine had sent a team of journalists; there were uptown-looking women hanging around, looking blasé, and men with gold necklaces trying to get in a word with some of the top competitors. You had the feeling in the lobby, and in some of the suites and the coffee shop and on the street in front of the hotel, that deals were being made here this year, that there were a lot of people around trying to get in on the ground floor while there still was one.

Late that morning a photo session was held on the mezzanine floor for the print journalists and, primarily, for George Snyder's video crew. Joe Weider, the first and biggest tenant on the ground floor, was there along with Sheila Herman, a writer for his magazines, and Susan Fry, a cool, willowy, chic woman who also works for Joe's magazines and is one of the leading organizers of women's bodybuilding. The head organizer, Doris Barrilleaux, was there too, being whispered to by Weider before the session began, dressed in an orange jumpsuit, her hard brown stomach showing.

One by one the contestants (or most of them; not all had been invited) came out and posed for the video crew, a dozen or so photographers and a small audience. Lynn Conkwright, who had already been photographed that morning running up the *Rocky* steps in front of the Philadelphia Public Library, looked perky and fit. Rachel McLish was smoother and visibly heavier than she had been the year before, but curvier too and radiant. Candy Csencsits looked like a lollypop, maybe, or a raspberry crush, in her hot-pink bikini and scarlet lipstick, her rich hair rampant and her gold and diamonds aglitter. At the end of the session George Snyder arranged all the women for a sweaty group shot with Doris Barrilleaux squatting and flexing in front of them, and then another with himself and Joe Weider posing with the bodybuilders like two happy anglers at either end of a string of caught fish.

Throughout the middle of the day the video crew filmed Ricky Wayne interviewing various contestants and organizers, and the interviews provided a kind of chorus to the other goings-on in the hotel, dealing as Ricky had them do with the use of drugs, the influence of men on women's bodybuilding, the question of what judges are and should be looking for, and the future of the sport.

Ricky Wayne: "Do you see a Miss Olympia winner as eventually becoming the Playboy ideal?"

Doris Barrilleaux and Rachel McLish: "Yes. Definitely."

Wayne: "What do you say to the people who say that all of this is unfeminine?"

Carolyn Cheshire: "There's nothing feminine about looking all soft and squishy."

Wayne: "You're more cut up this year, aren't you, Georgia?"

Georgia Miller Fudge: "Yes, I am. I think it's beautiful to see the separation between the muscles—that's what I wanted this year."

Wayne: "Why do you do this?"

Fudge: "Because I want to feel good about myself."

Wayne: "And how do your women friends react to you?"

Fudge: "I don't have many women friends. My husband is my friend."

At four-thirty Doris Barrilleaux called a competitors' meeting to discuss the state of women's bodybuilding on this the eve of its second annual professional championships. The meeting was conducted by Doris, Susan Fry, and Kim Cassidy, a pleasant midwestern woman with a straightforward air about her who serves as

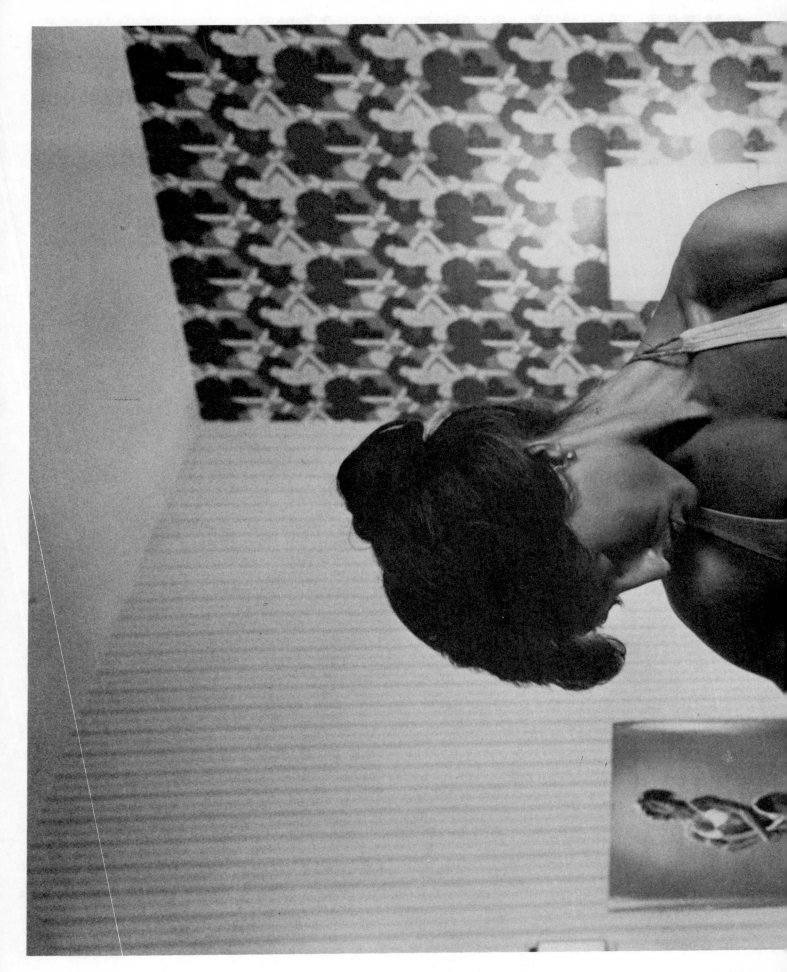

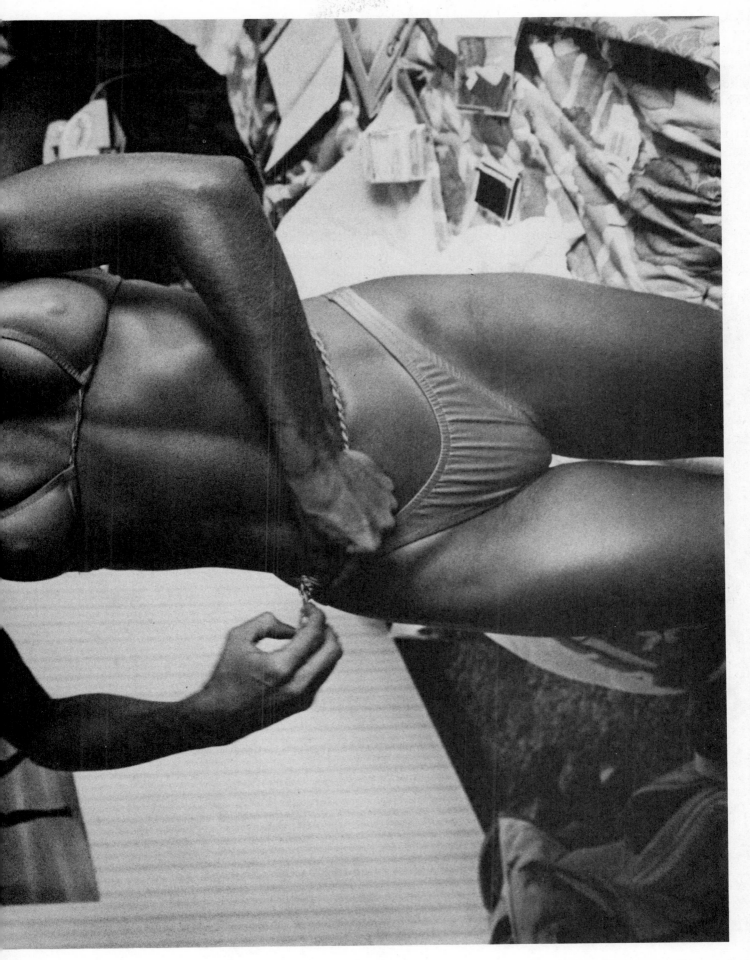

Rachel McLish, Philadelphia, 1981

Treasurer and Sanction Secretary of the American Federation of Women Bodybuilders, the governing body for amateur female bodybuilding competitors in the United Sates. The president of this organization—which is the amateur equivalent of the professional Women's Committee of the International Federation of Body Builders, chaired by Doris Barrilleaux—is, unsurprisingly, Doris Barrilleaux. And the general secretary for both organizations is Susan Fry. The two organizations sanctioned roughly two hundred female bodybuilding competitions around the country in 1981, from small city and town competitions to state championships to the top national contests (the Women's America and USA for amateurs, the World Championships for pro-am, and the Miss Olympia for professionals).

Doris and Susan and Kim sat on the stage in the hotel's ballroom and took questions and comments from their constituency. The women talked about the importance of presentation—the combination of free poses which showcases the individual results of their training—and agreed that they would like for it to count for one-third of what the judges judged, along with muscularity and symmetry. They worried at length about the use of drugs, particularly steroids, and wondered whether competitors should be given drug tests after competitions the way Olympic athletes are, or lie-detector tests, or should be certified regularly as drug-clean by clinics around the country. There was a lot of discussion on the character of compulsory poses,

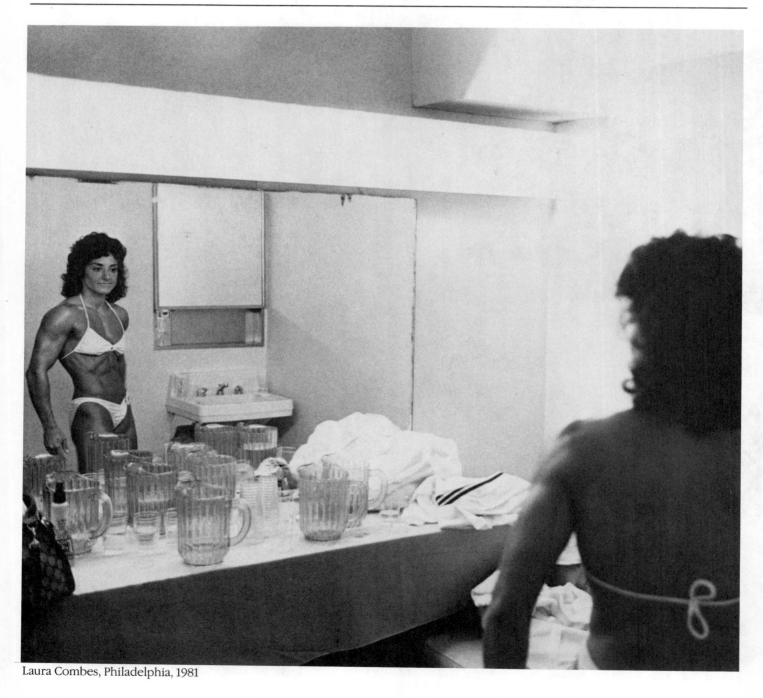

Laura Combes, Philadelphia, 1981

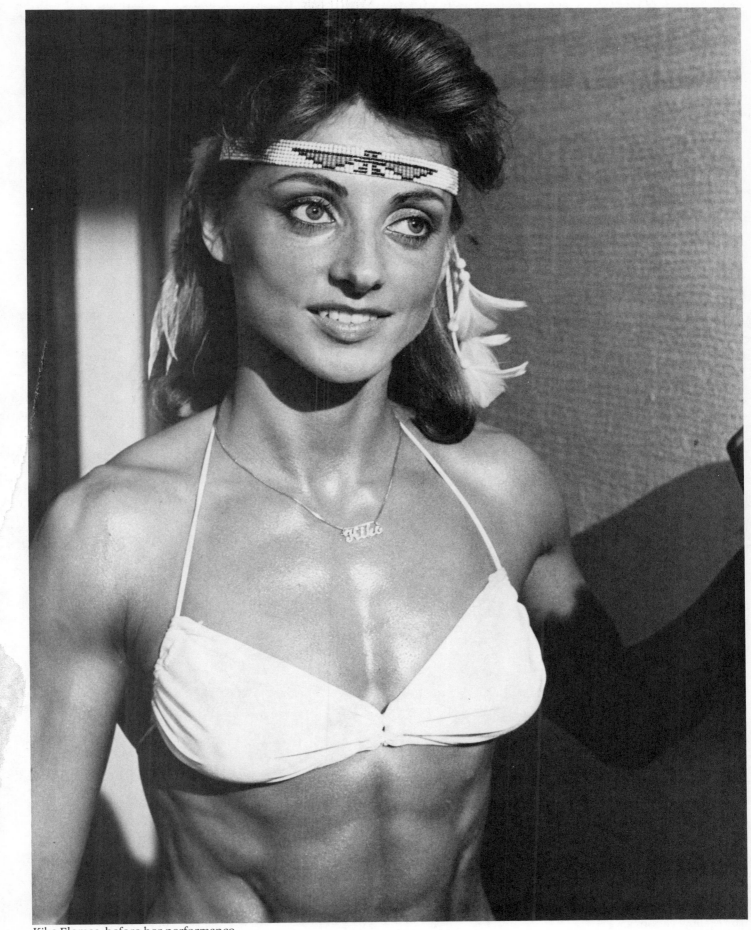

Kike Elomaa, before her performance

"I talked with Bill Pearl and he said there's only one way for the sport to go, to achieve size and shape and definition, just like the men. It doesn't mean you have to look like a man, it just means you have to go for it. How can you judge a sport without going to the max? That's what it's all about, seeing how far you can go."
—Laura Combes

mostly directed at feminizing (since none of the big-muscle women entered in the competition were at the meeting) and standardizing them. And that discussion led to a general and hotly felt condemnation of certain men, among them a number of writers, who in their efforts to impose male ideas and aesthetics on female bodybuilding were, in the view of these women, seriously damaging the sport by championing the wrong things (i.e., big muscles) and the wrong people (i.e., the female competitors who have them).

There was no discussion about how to make women's bodybuilding more acceptable to the general public, how to build a larger audience for it, how to draw more favorable national publicity, or how to improve the often lackluster theatricality of the competitions. It

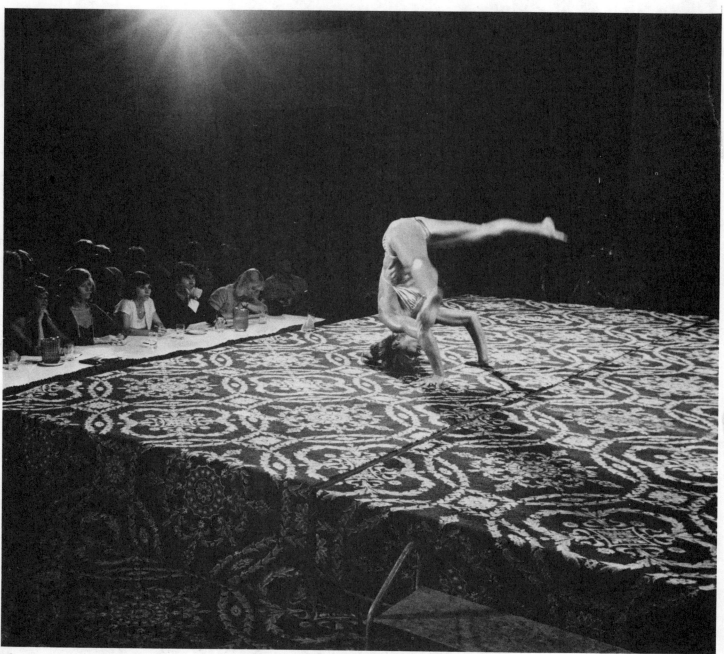

The Evening Performance

was clear that the women gathered there in the ball-room were conservatives, more concerned, for the time being anyway, with keeping at bay the big-muscle forces, both inside and outside the sport, than with the sort of overall expansion and improvement that male bodybuilding had undergone in the past eight years. And if the meeting had a sort of sorority-house, coffee-klatch sweetness and sisterliness to it, it also had a corresponding feel of cliquishness, an evangelical, us-against-them tone.

Laura Combes was not there. But you had the strong impression that if she had been, with her big shoulders and her independent ideas, the meeting might have been more productive.

"I actually feel like if that's their goal [to develop big muscles], then they should actually compete with men in the lightweight categories, you know? Because if you wapped off their heads they'd look like a man, so why not enter the men's contests?"
—Lynn Conkwright

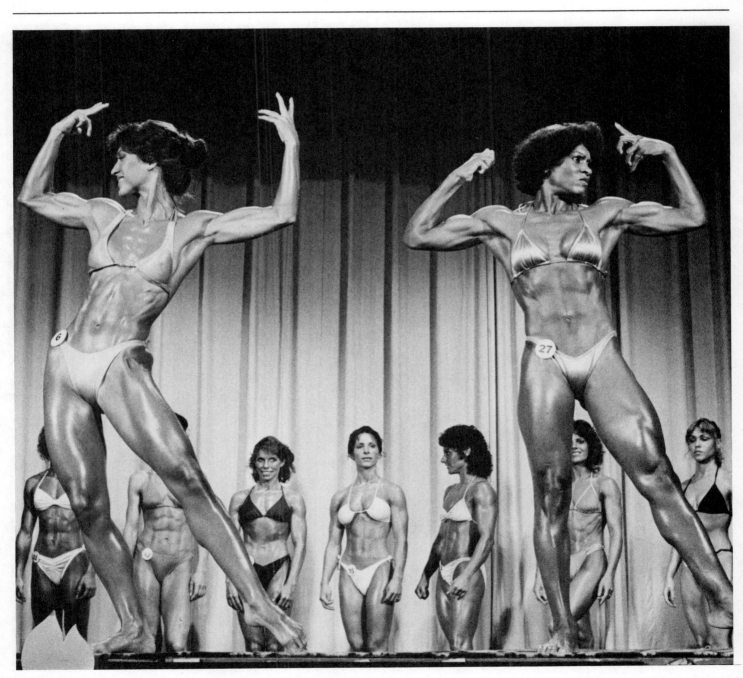

Prejudging

"The best part about it is when the little kids come up and say, 'Hey, I've been training.' I say, 'Oh, you have?' And they say they can lift a hundred and fifty pounds. You got a little kid like this standing there and you're thinking, God, I could never have said that when I was a kid. If nothing else, we're knocking down some trees for some people behind us."
—Laura Combes

Laura Combes was twenty-seven years old in the summer of 1981. Originally from New York City, she now lives in Tampa, Florida, where she started weight training eleven years before for rehabilitation after knee surgery. Like Lynn Conkwright and Rachel McLish and many other women bodybuilders, she has always been athletic. She was captain of the 1972 national champion University of South Florida water-ski team. After college she played five years of rugby, and was on the team that won the 1979 national female rugby championship in Chicago. In that same year she won her first bodybuilding title, Miss Tampa. The television program *Real People* filmed that contest, and when the show was aired Laura and her big muscles became an overnight national controversy. Later that year she won

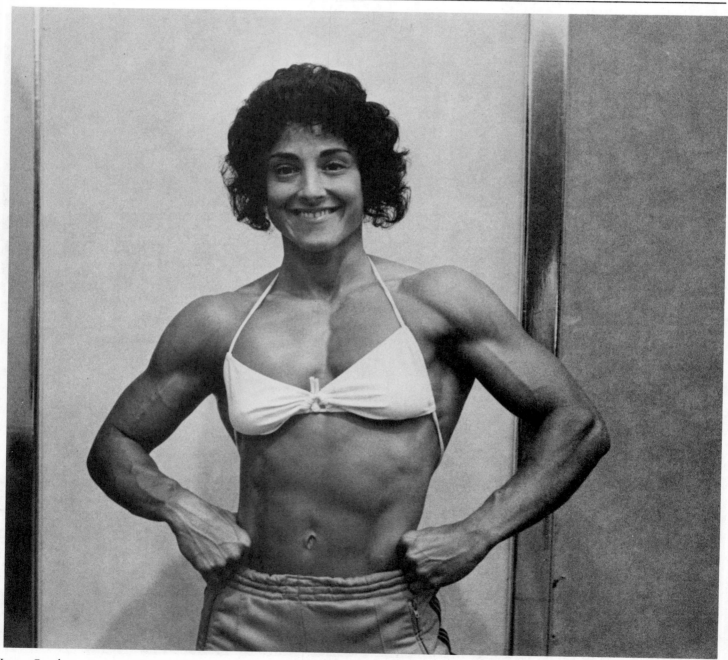

Laura Combes

the Miss Northwest Florida contest, and in 1980 the Miss Florida title, and then the amateur American Women's Bodybuilding Championship in Los Angeles. But increasingly, through this string of victories, Laura found herself occupying the less populated and popular side of women's bodybuilding's widening central dispute—and to a lot of people, not just occupying it, but *representing* it. Through 1979 and '80 she became, without really trying to, one-half of an argument. She came to stand for something more than herself, and whenever she entered a contest that something entered with her, making each competition for her not only a contest between individual bodies but between aesthetic ideals as well.

Laura Combes is a *muscular* woman, muscular not in the athletic, ballet-dancer, gymnast way that Lynn Conkwright and Rachel McLish are muscular, but in a way that is qualitatively different from that. To say that she looks like a man, as has been said, is both unkind and untrue. But she does not, dressed in a bikini, look like a run-of-the-mill woman either. She is five feet two inches tall and weighs one hundred twenty pounds. Her shoulders are wide and muscular, and her arms actually bulge. There is very little hourglass curve between her ribcage and her hips, and her waist is hard and ridged. Unlike Rachel McLish, she is not traditionally pretty, or traditionally "cute" like Lynn Conkwright. She has a strong face with wide cheekbones, a sharply aquiline nose and large, dark, no-nonsense eyes. She is a smart woman from an upper-middle-

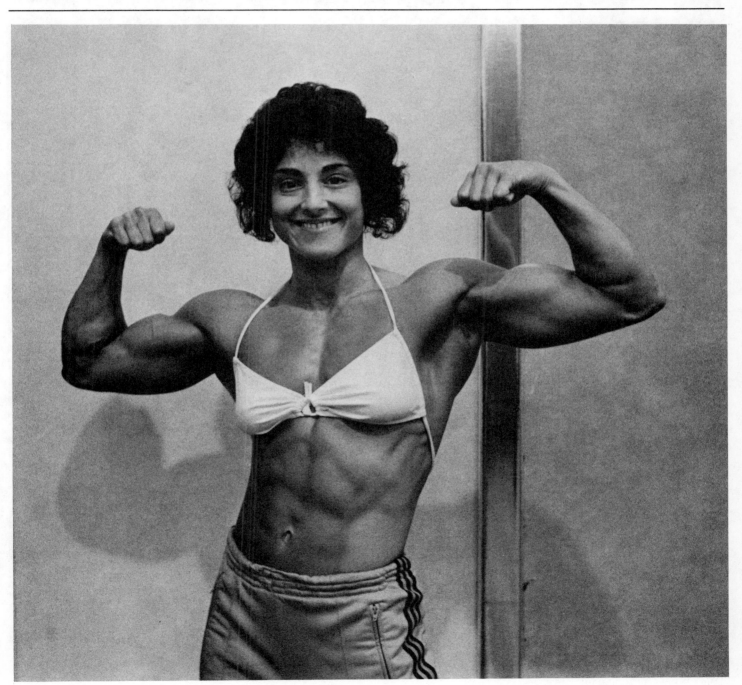

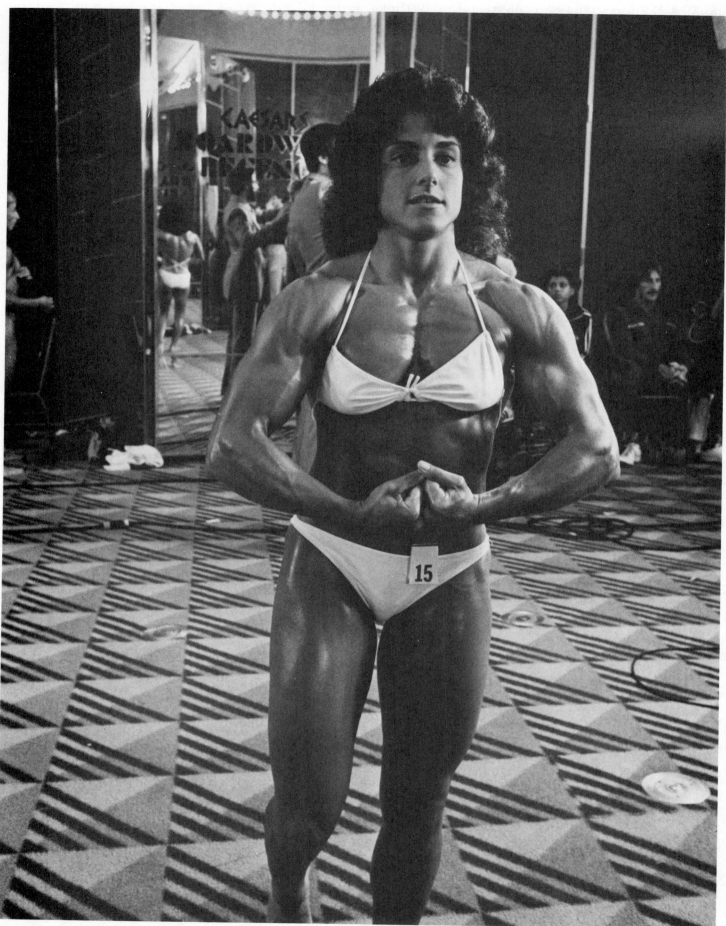

Laura Combes, pumping up

"In Europe we don't like the big muscular girls. We think they are like men without mustache."
—Kimmo Elomaa

class background who has been a top athlete for most of her life, a woman used to doing and getting what she wants, and nowhere about her is there any of the slightly dazed, Tammy-like quality of some of the other women in the sport.

I talked to her in the morning of the day of the Miss Olympia contest. I asked her first how her year had gone and, since along with Rachel and maybe Lynn, she is one of the very few women to make a living at bodybuilding, how that living had been. She said she had traveled a lot and had gotten a lot of guest-posing shots around the country because she hadn't over-priced herself. She gets around seven hundred dollars plus expenses for guest posing, and either half the attendance gate or three hundred dollars for a semi-

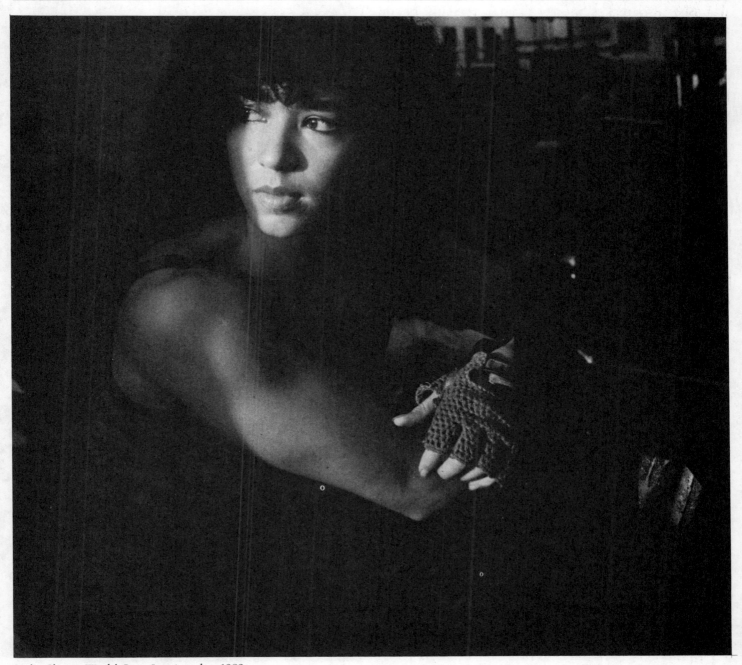

Lydia Cheng, World Gym, Los Angeles, 1983

83

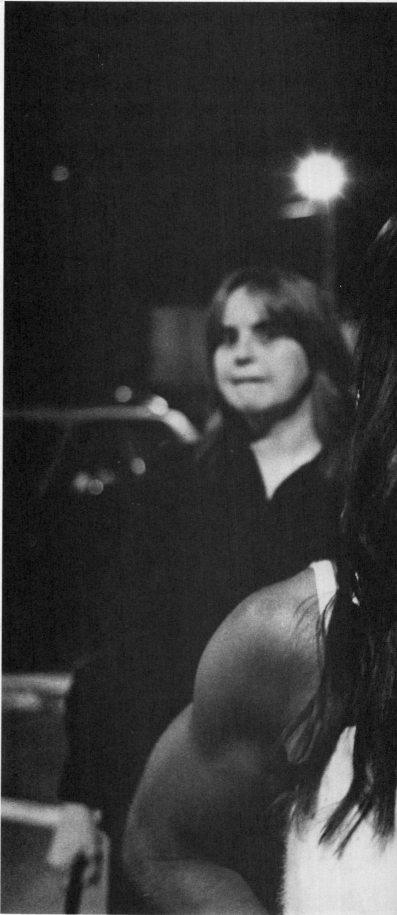

nar. She also makes money from a recently begun mail-order business selling training courses and photographs and T-shirts, and occasionally from endorsements. I asked her if she had made, say, thirty-five thousand dollars this year. "Oh no, not that much," she said. "I'm making a living, let's put it that way." (By comparison, Rachel McLish, who is much more in demand as a product endorser, claims to have earned around forty thousand dollars in 1980, "just here and there, not really trying, not really pushing.")

Laura earns what money she does because of her media exposure, which despite her not yet having won a major professional contest, has been at least the equal of any woman in the sport. Why, I wondered, did she think that was so? Well, she said, for one thing she was more muscular than most of the other women, and that made for good copy. And for another, "I always do what I want to do, regardless of what judges are looking for, because I feel this is an art form and I should be able to express myself however I like. For instance, when they said you can't clench your fists when you pose, I said baloney and did it anyway."

Does it make her feel any less feminine to be as muscular as she is? "No. Because I think femininity is inside you. It's a state of mind, and being a lady and acting like a lady come from inside your personality. Having a little bit different equipment to walk around with has nothing to do with it. Also, being strong makes me feel self-sufficient. My self-esteem is up and that's like part of a new era that has begun for women in general. If a woman wants to do something now, she can do it. Don't talk about it, don't crab about it, just do it."

And what did she have to say about the big issue, the issue that this contest, and most others until it is settled, was likely only to exacerbate—the muscles-versus-pretty-bodies issue which had affected her as much as anyone and remained the hard knot at the center of female bodybuilding?

As it happened, Laura had quite a bit to say on that

Rachel with Karen and Wayne DeMilia, Philadelphia, 1981

84

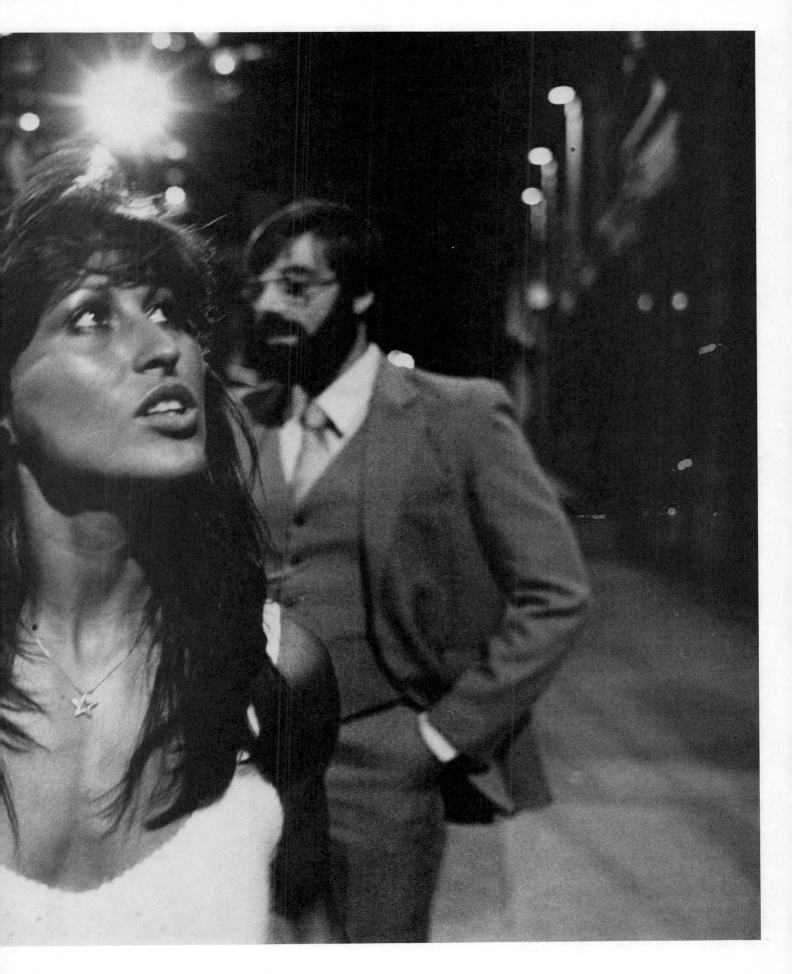

issue: "I think the leaders of this sport are holding the sport back because they're trying to keep muscularity out of it, and trying to say what women should look like. I think they should be asking, what *can* women look like? Let 'em go, free it up, and we'll see what's going on here, and then judge—don't start holding us back before it even begins. We haven't even started to know what our whole potential is yet." And: "If all these women keep holding back because they have to look softer, that's not *training*. How can you do a sport without going to the max? That's what it's all about, seeing how far you can go." And: "Eventually people are going to get used to it. The norm is going to be the muscular woman. You see this other stuff everywhere. You see models, you see ballet dancers. I don't think a

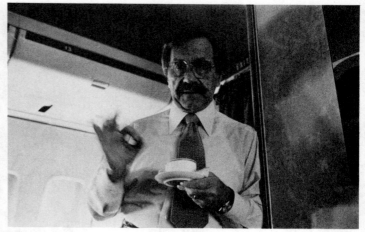

Joe Weider

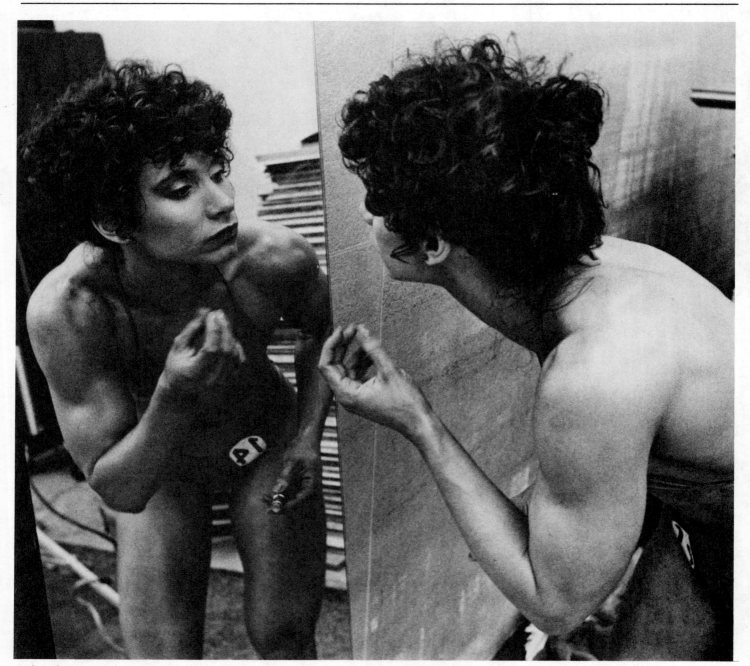

Deborah Diana, Atlantic City

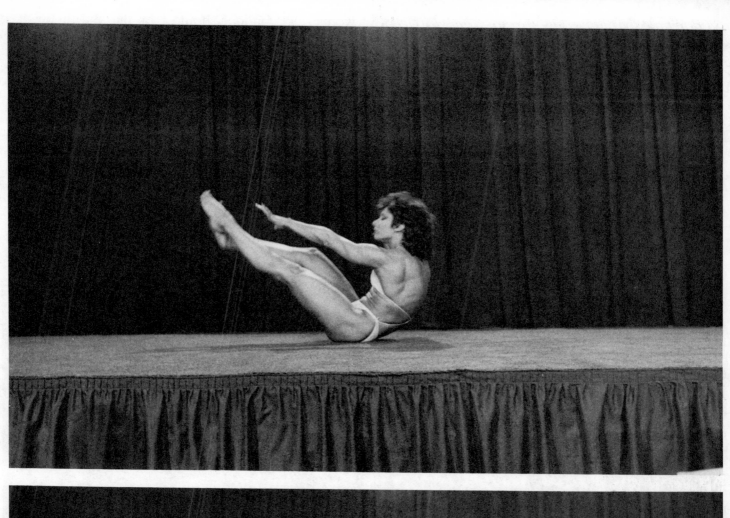

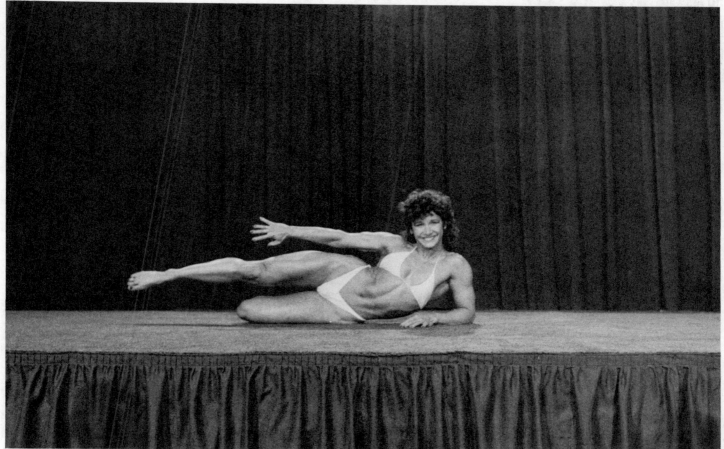

Deborah Diana, Atlantic City

"I don't put the blame on these girls themselves who are taking steroids. I put the blame on the coaches and trainers out there who are looking for shortcuts, ways to add to their own prestige, who get these women started on drugs. It's stupid. Women using steroids is a shortcut to nowhere."
—Johnny Peebles III, Director of Strength and Conditioning, Jewish Community Center, Birmingham, Alabama

woman bodybuilder should look like a gymnast or a dancer—she should look like a bodybuilder. Just like the men. You have male gymnasts who have great bodies, male dancers, but bodybuilders don't look like either one of them. I think there *should* be a difference."

Finally I asked her what she thought of her chances to win this year's Miss Olympia. Laura shrugged, then smiled. "This is a subjective sport anyway and the judges sometimes . . . well, the judging has to come a long ways too. You just have to take your lumps. A lot of these women who started the sport were not athletes. They were not used to losing. As an athlete you have to take winning and losing, and I've lost some big things in my life, so losing just makes me want to come

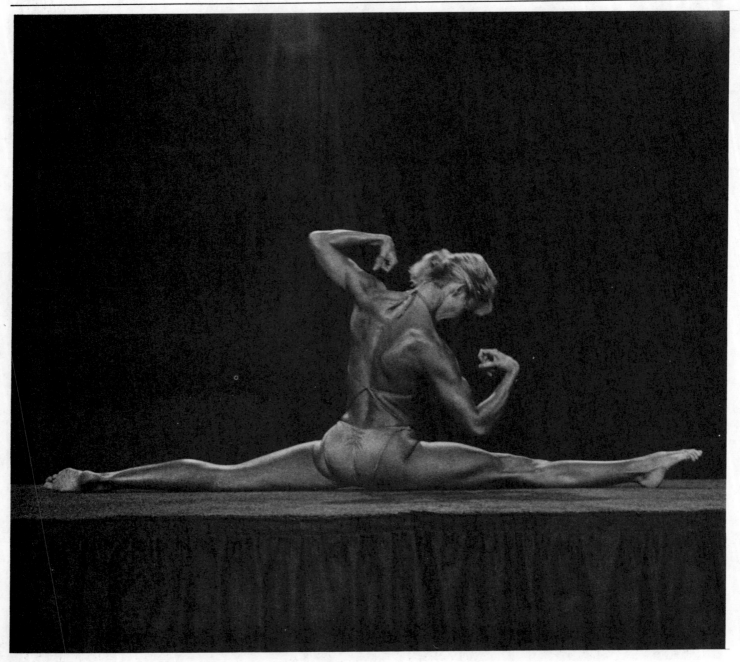

Shelly Gruwell

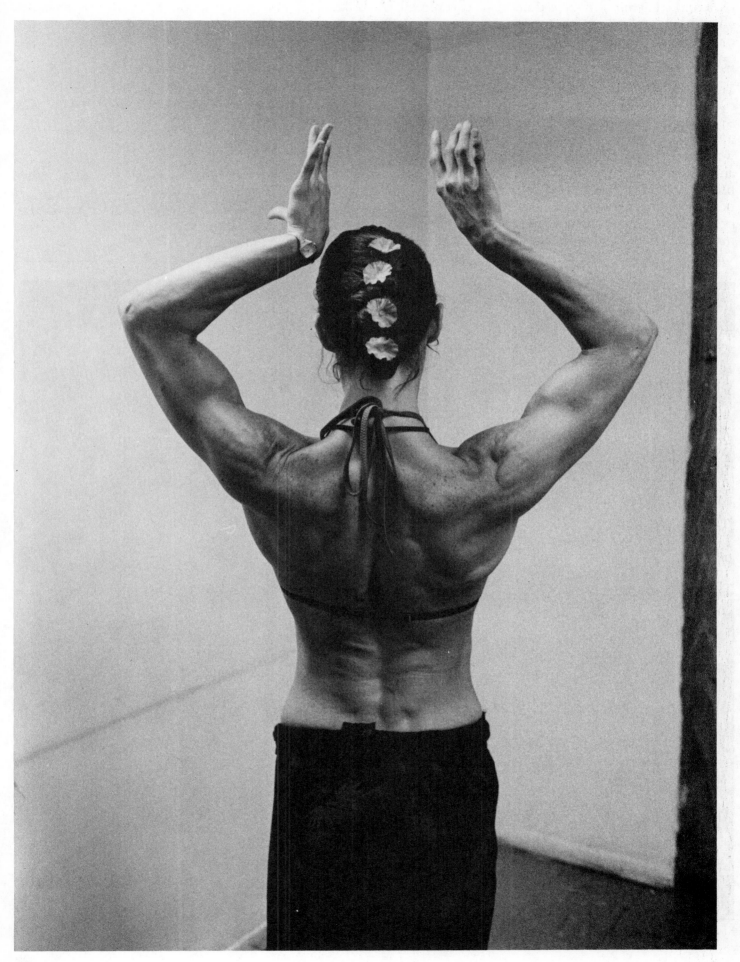

back and try it again . . . . If I don't do it this time, I'm going to come back next year, and I'm going to keep coming back until I get it right. Or until the judges do."

There was a dark horse entered in the 1981 Olympia contest, a woman on whom practically no one at the Sheraton had set eyes until the prejudging. Until then it was generally expected that the real competition would be between Rachel McLish, Lynn Conkwright and Laura Combes, with Rachel, the reigning titlist, probably the favorite. But as soon as the twenty competitors came out on stage as a group to begin the prejudging, gleaming with baby oil, tanned, and grinning for all they were worth, it was evident that there

"I like it all. Rachel's my favorite, but none of them are too muscular out there today. I thought it was all feminine."

"Their skin, they're all firm, from the backs of their legs where girls have a lot of problems. I think these girls could blow away your normal girls on the beach, and they look better in jeans."

"It turns me on to a certain degree."

"It doesn't turn me on. No, definitely. It's just nice to watch."

—Three young men from New York City at the 1981 Miss Olympia contest, their first women's bodybuilding competition

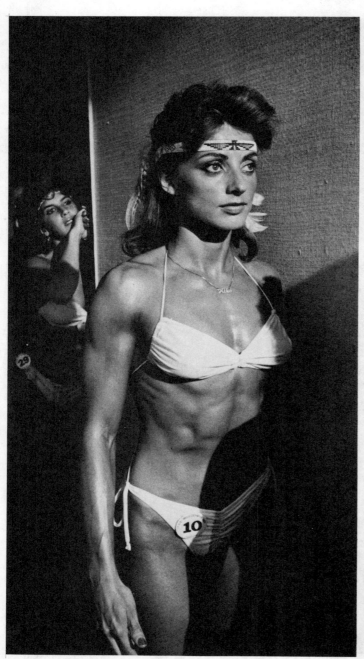

Kike Elomaa

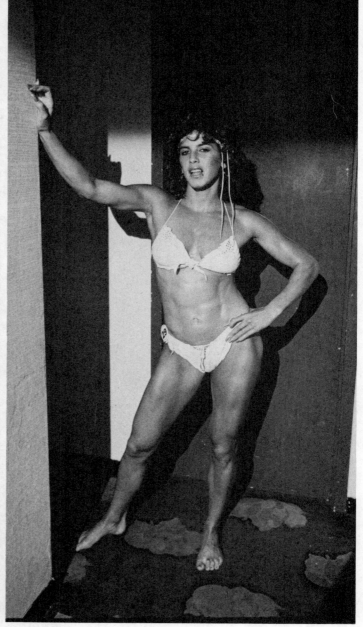

Kyle Newman

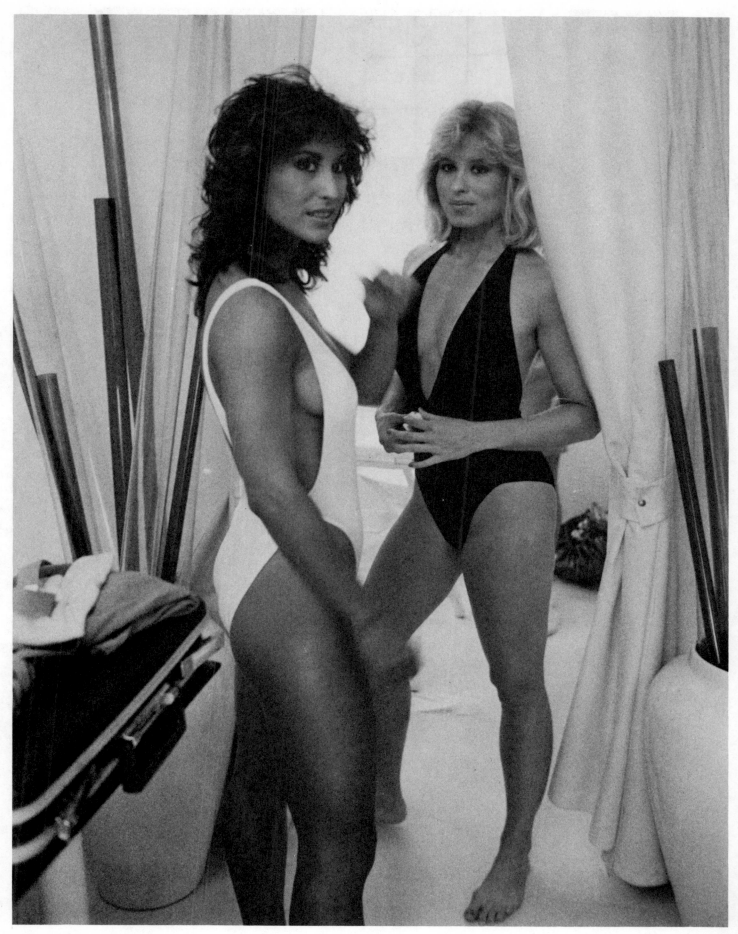

Rachel and Winnie Gardner

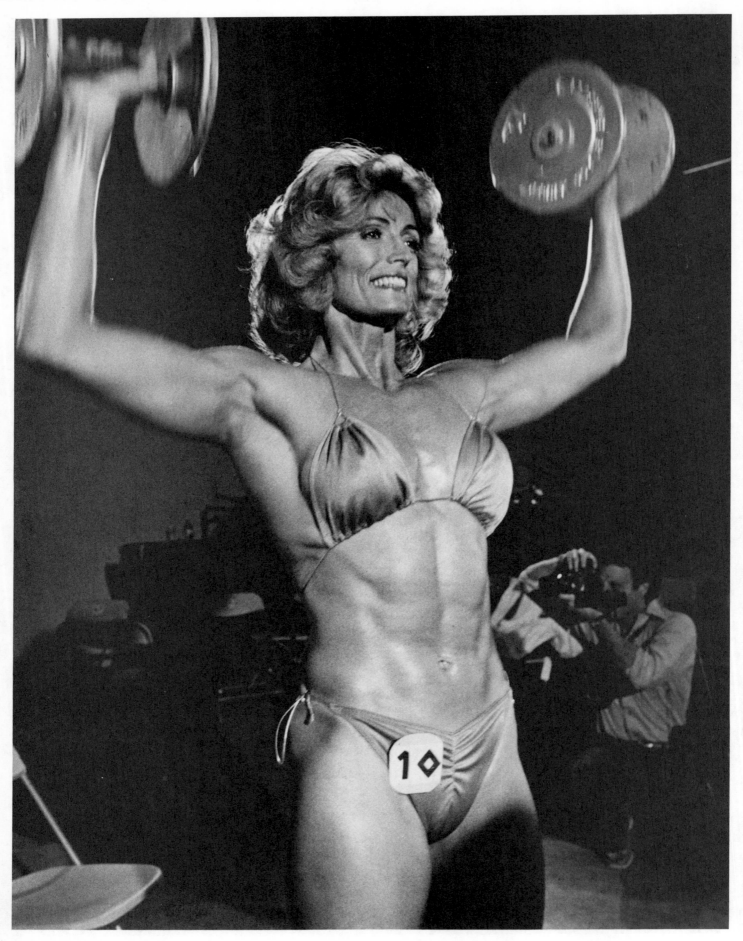

Dr. Lynn Pirie, Las Vegas, 1982

was one other very serious contender. Her name was Kike Elomaa, and though a month earlier she had won the middle-weight female bodybuilding title of the first World Games Competition held in Santa Clara, California, she was so unheralded an entry at the Miss Olympia that she was not even listed in the contest's program.

Kike and her husband-trainer, Kimmo, are Finnish. They kept very much to themselves and, for the most part, out of sight at the Sheraton, and so she came as a shock to everyone at the prejudging who had not seen her in Santa Clara. She is a beautifully shaped woman, with the same kind of eye-catching finish to her body that Rachel McLish has. Your eye tended to return to her in the prejudging lineup and to linger on her. In

Finland before she began bodybuilding she was a sprinter and long jumper, and her legs were spectacular, fully muscled and delicately proportioned. Though her upper body was not as muscular as Laura Combes's —except for her abdominals, which were as cleanly separated and visually surprising on a woman as Auby Paulick's had been the year before—it was developed well beyond simple tone, and her face was pretty and proudly expressionless.

It is difficult to look objectively at women bodybuilders in the prejudging lineup. Much more than with the men, there is a cattle-auction, cheesecake feel to it which is almost always reinforced by their expressions. You notice the expressions on the faces of male bodybuilders only when they are embarrassing them-

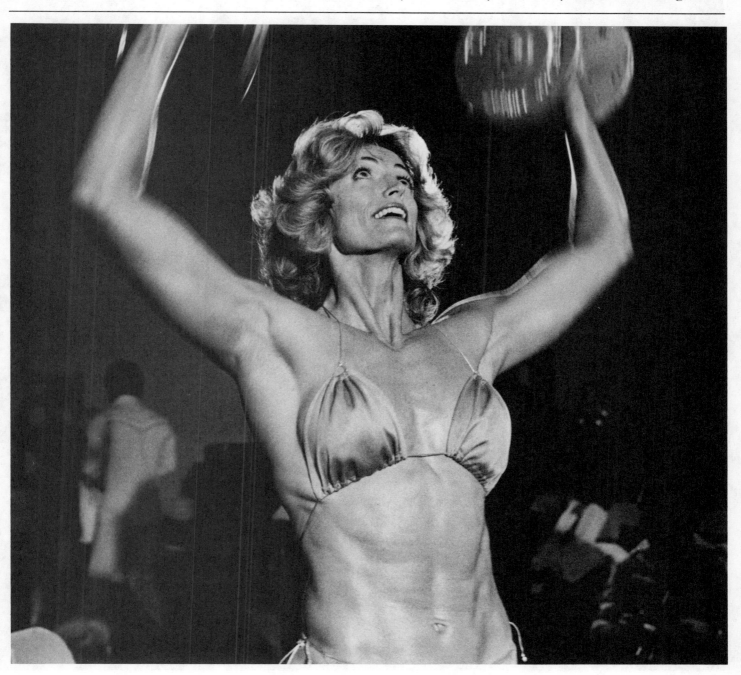

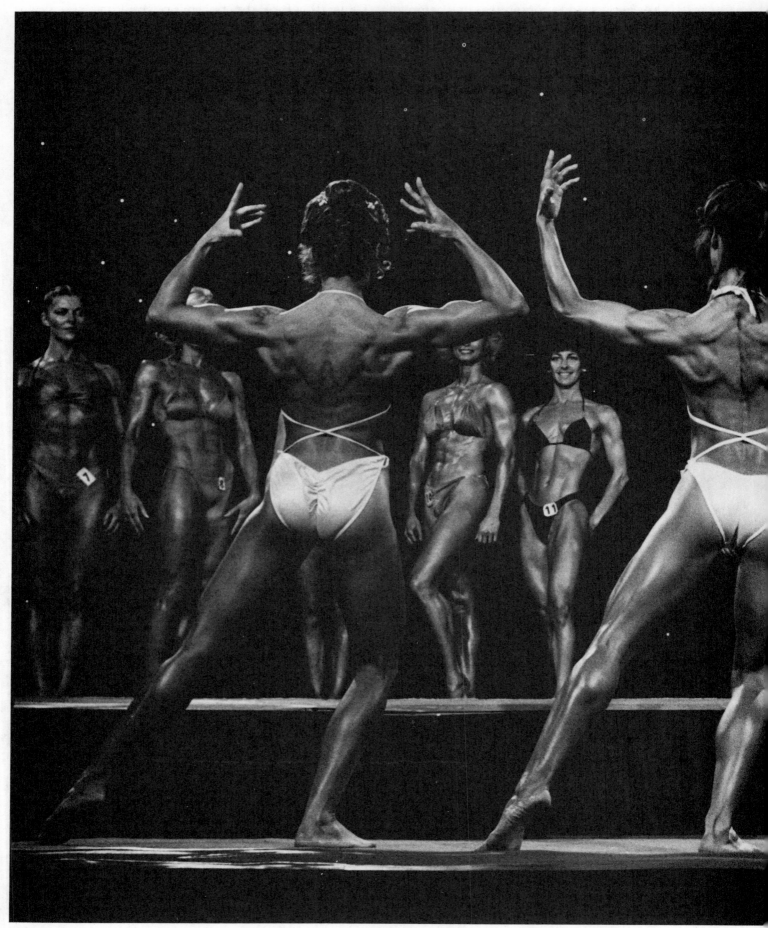

Las Vegas, 1982

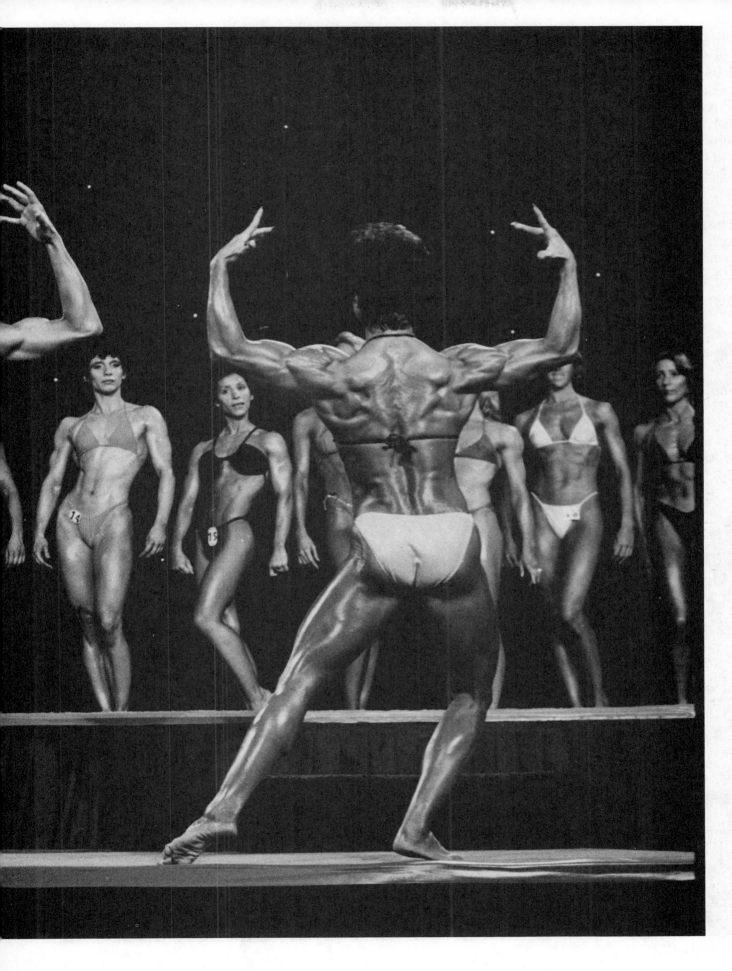

selves, when they are out of shape or posing poorly, and even then there is very little in their faces to read. The women tend to show whatever they are feeling, and watching them, without the visually fascinating, big, complex muscles of the men to hold your attention, you tend to feel along with them: anger, envy, embarrassment and, most common of all, a touching eagerness to please.

Without much muscle, Donna Frame, the former Oakland Raider cheerleader, looked very eager to please. Ellen Davis didn't; she looked mad. Kyle Newman, a former Miss Long Island, looked tempestuous and lusty. Lynn Conkwright looked fresh and eager, as though she had just come inside to a big vegetarian breakfast after feeding the stock. Laura Combes looked

combative, and Rachel McLish, flashing her ingratiating Miss America smile at the judges, looked confident, even a little imperial. But Kike Elomaa's cool Finnish face was absolutely expressionless. She stood in the lineup with her shoulders held back, her little bobbed head high, listening to Kimmo shout out instructions and encouragement in Finnish from the audience, and looking coolly up at the ceiling, waiting for things to begin.

After Round One of the prejudging, the nonposing round in which symmetry and proportion are judged, and before Round Two—in which overall muscularity is judged in a series of seven compulsory poses which, because they are taken from the men and designed to articulate strength and power, looked diminished and

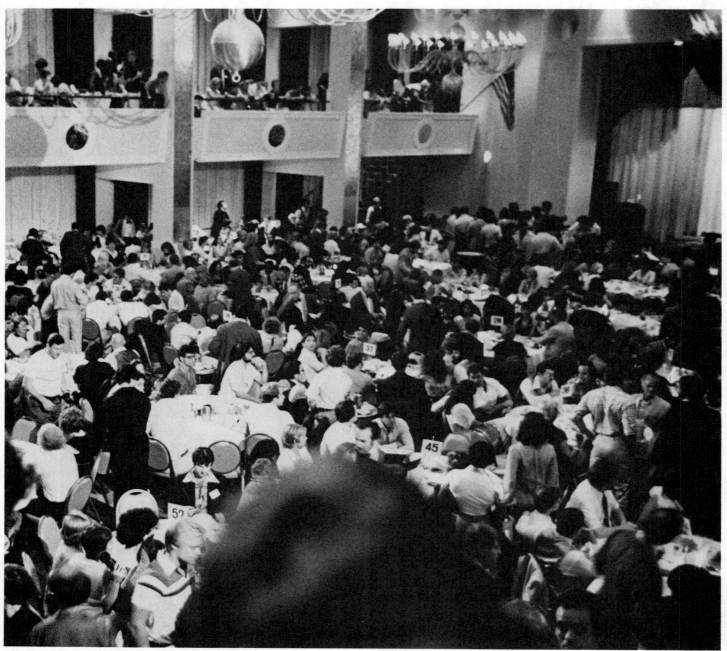

The Evening Performance, Philadelphia, 1981

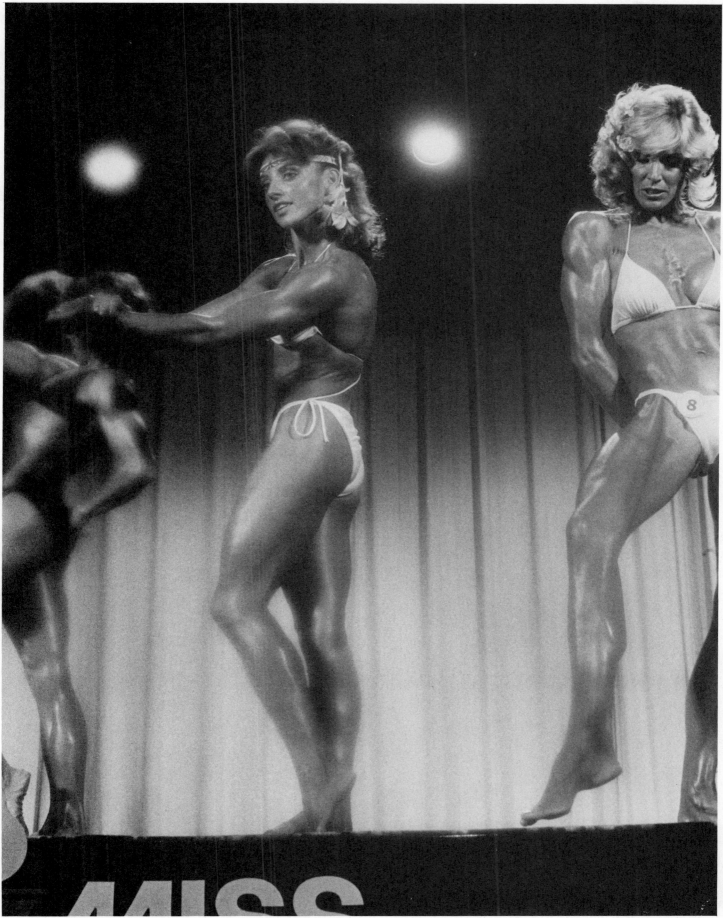

Poseoff

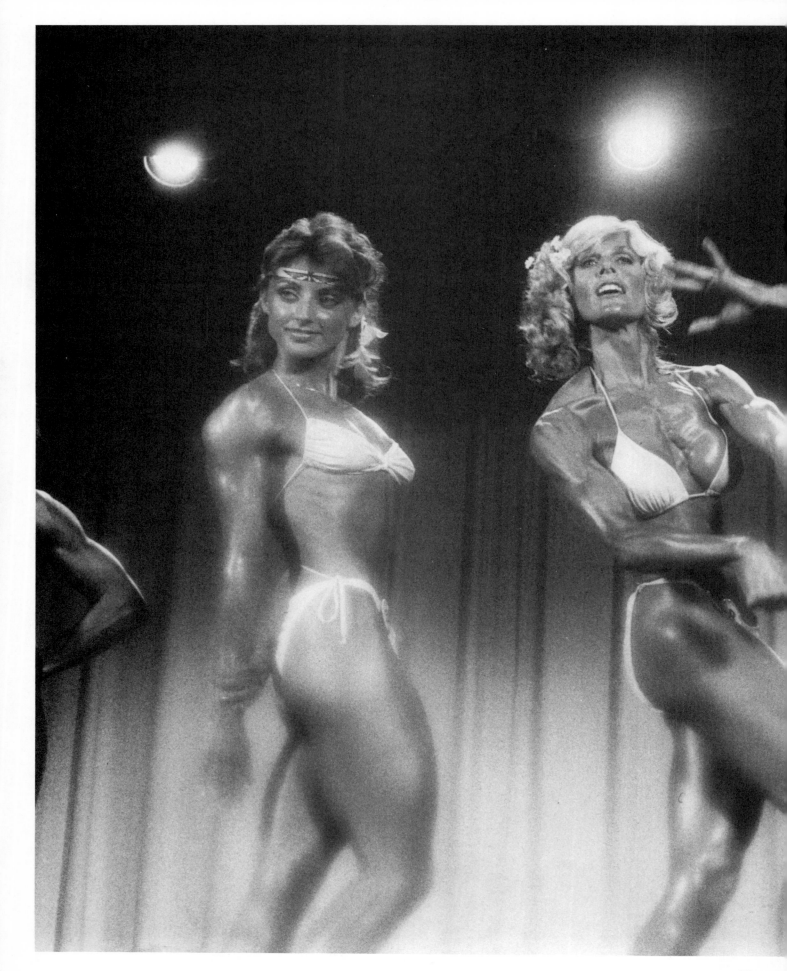

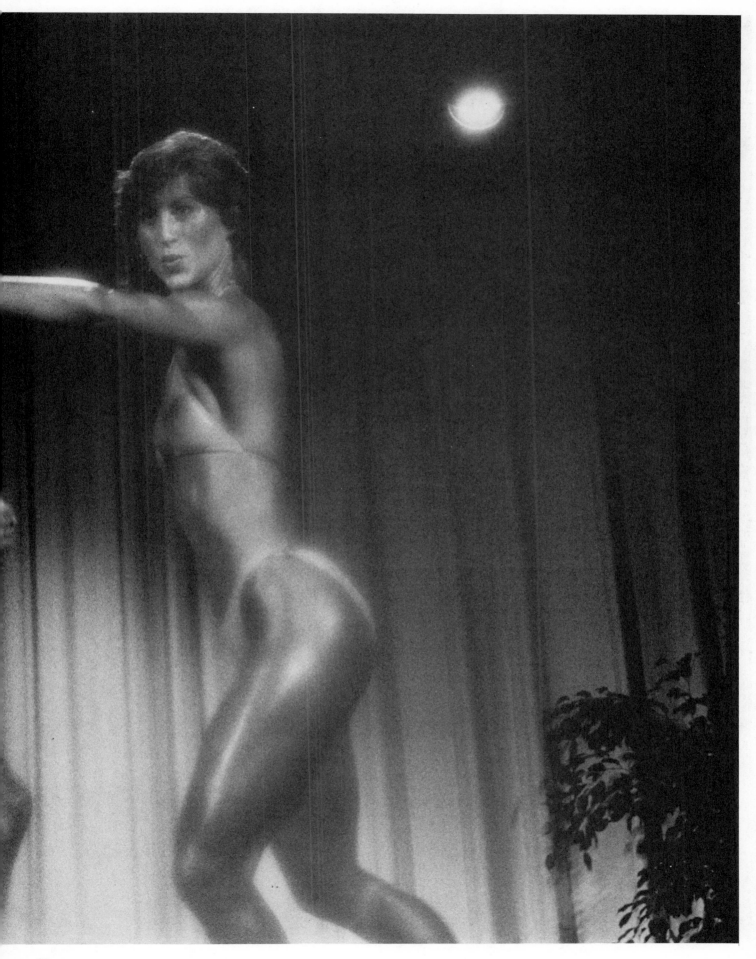

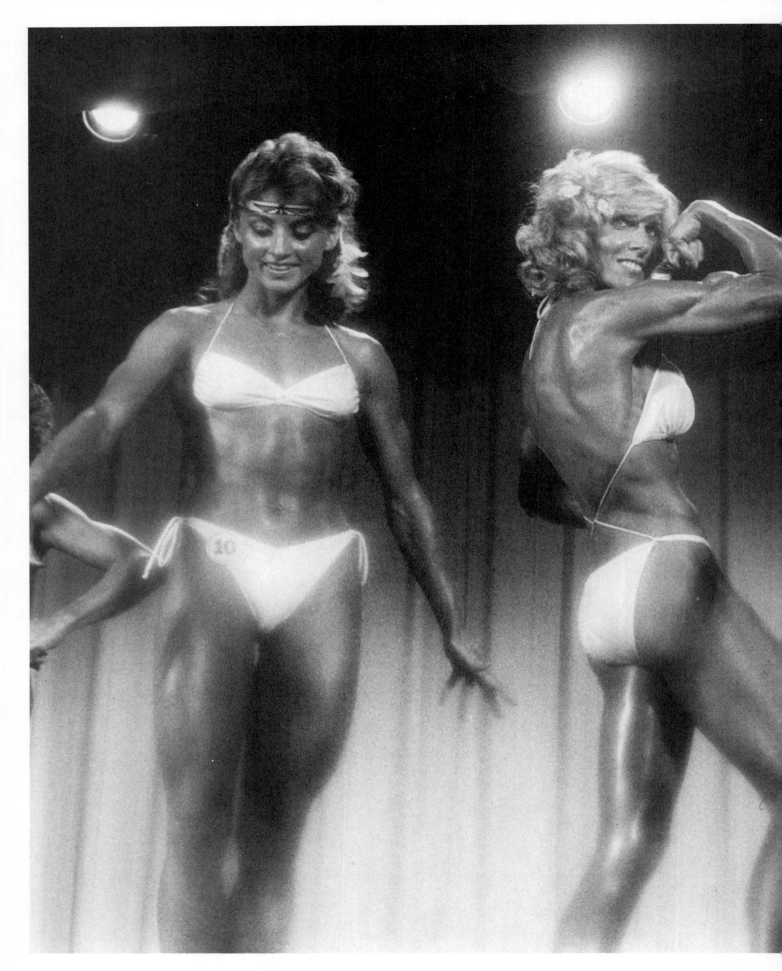

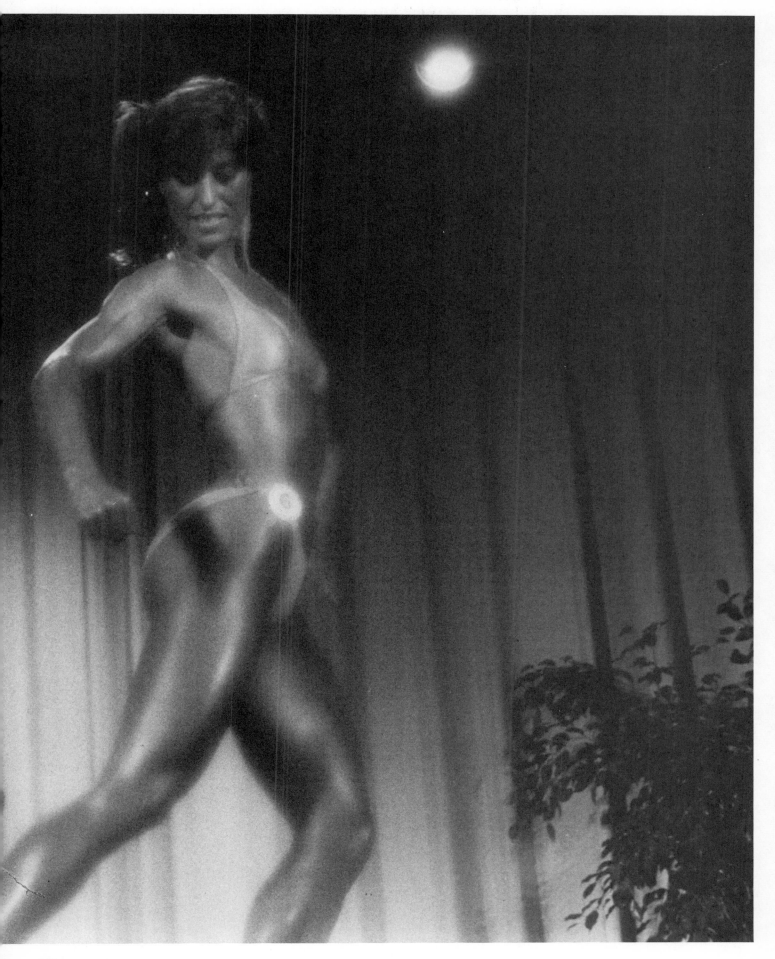

often downright silly when struck by women—there was a five-minute break. During it I asked a well-known and controversial women's bodybuilding writer what he thought about the competition so far.

"The Finnish girl ought to win it but she won't," he said.

"Why not?"

"Because this is a completely controlled contest, don't you know that?"

"Controlled by whom and to what end?" I asked him.

"By the forces that be," he said, "and to make money, of course, off of women's bodybuilding. The Finn isn't as marketable as Rachel. It's as simple as that," said the writer. "She can't win."

Backstage, just before the nighttime show of the Miss Olympia contest, Laura Combes is walking around flexing her shoulders and doing one-legged calf raises. The mood is friendly and there is none of the sullen gloom of backstage immediately before a men's contest. Lynn Conkwright, with a blue flower in her hair, walks into an anteroom and looks at her gleaming, bikinied body in a mirror. She flexes a thigh.

"Get that little sucker out there," says Kyle Newman, studying the clear deep groove between two of Lynn's thigh muscles. "Jesus. I don't even *have* that."

Out front in the ballroom a dressed-up audience of around two thousand people is finishing dinner; in front of each of them sits a piece of apple pie topped with a slice of Velveeta cheese. *Tout le monde* of body-

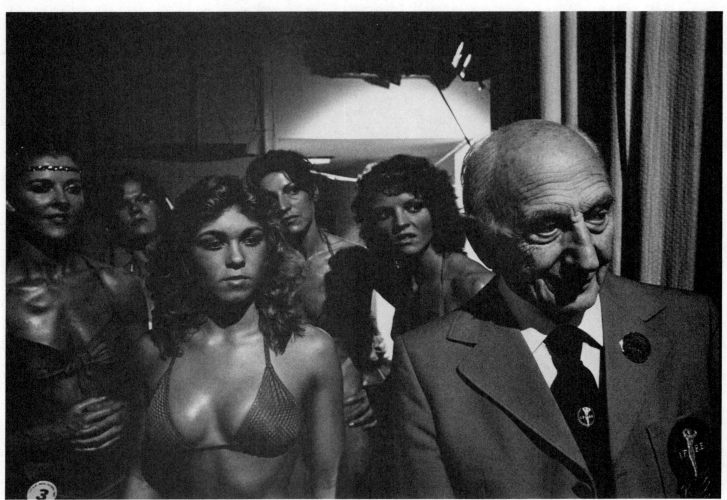

Oscar State

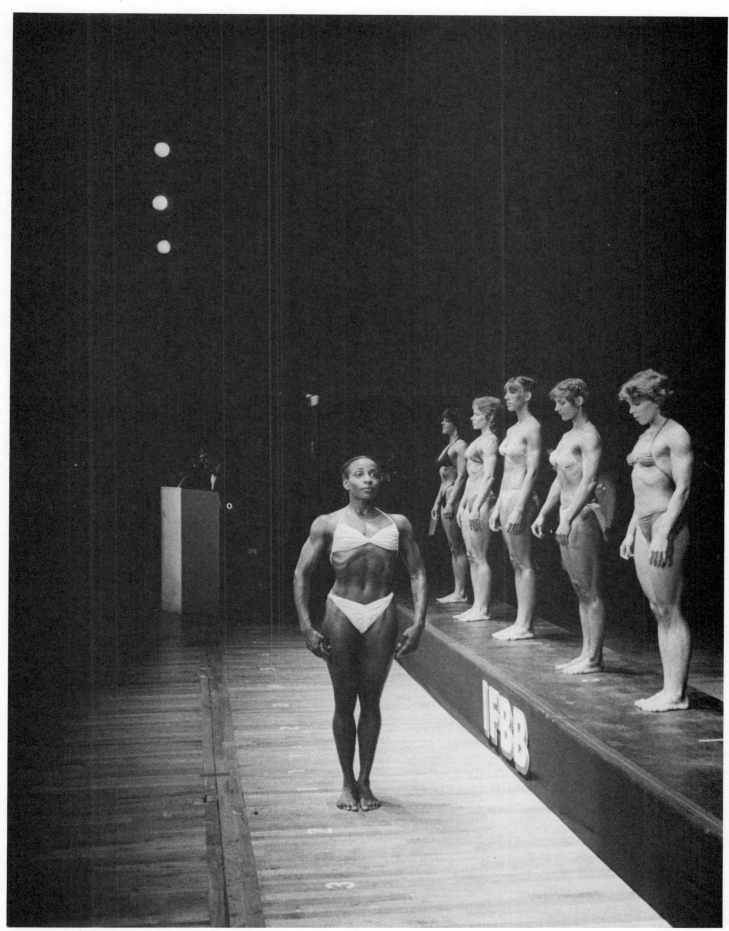

Carla Dunlap, Prejudging, New York

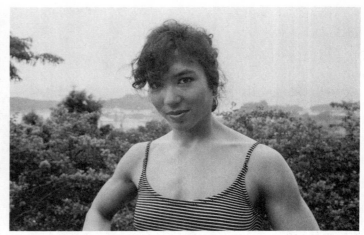

Lydia Cheng, Singapore

building is out there, and most of the women backstage peer out at the tables from time to time, their faces registering exactly what they are feeling. Kike Elomaa doesn't look out at the audience at all, and her husband is not backstage. She wears a rawhide headband with a big feather, and her face, as she stands off by herself in the wings, is indrawn and calm.

Danny Padilla starts the show with a witty, massive posing routine, and brings the house down. Earlier that day Kyle Newman, the smoky ex–Miss Long Island, had asked me if I thought Danny had any money. She held up her hand and looked at a diamond stud set into one of her long red fingernails. I said I doubted if he had a lot. "Comfortable," she said. "Do you think he's comfortable?" "Are you looking for a guy with money, then," I asked. "Well . . . ," she said and shrugged. "I mean if you can't help me, for God's sake don't hinder me."

Kyle is dressed in a buckskin bikini, with a piece of leather in her black hair. She looks sultry and terrific, like some Rodeo Drive producer's idea of Hiawatha. When Padilla is finished out front, the gnomish little old English bodybuilding bigwig, Oscar State, who is tonight the official vote counter and with Doris Barrilleaux one of the two head judges, takes over, wearing a hideously bright red jacket. He introduces the master of ceremonies, and the show is underway.

Wayne DeMilia, organizer of the Grand Prix men's bodybuilding circuit and one of the most intelligent people in the sport, is coordinating things backstage. He had told me earlier that he had his doubts about the future of women's bodybuilding—that he wondered about the ability of the contests, without the big-muscle magic of the men's shows, to continue to draw crowds after the novelty had worn off. He had said too that he believed the use of steroids and other drugs among the women was growing (though he and others have estimated that that use is probably confined to five percent or less of the roughly one thousand to fifteen hundred registered female bodybuilding competitors), and that if it spread further it would kill the sport stone dead. In the meantime, though, Wayne DeMilia skillfully directs contestants from the dressing room to the hallway to the stage.

Waiting their turns in the hallway, Rachel pulls on a rope, Kike does a set of quiet, absorbed calf-raises, and Lynn sits on a step, her knees bouncing. Women around them are doing push-ups off the walls. As each new performance begins, the waiting women move their bare feet and legs to the music on stage, and occasionally step into the wings to watch the routine.

In the dressing room other competitors oil themselves, stretch and check poses in front of a mirror, and chat. Rachel, Candy Csencsits and Ellen Davis are lounging with a water pitcher and glasses and singing along to "Nobody Does It Better," the music to Georgia Miller Fudge's routine on stage. The music stops, and after a moment Georgia walks into the dressing room sobbing. Some people, after the prejudging, had told her that she looked too muscular and it had ruined the show for her tonight. Rachel, Candy and Ellen console her, Rachel with her arm around Georgia's wide, sinewy shoulders.

Rachel herself has a good new routine, performed with much more energy and commitment than last year and to better music. As usual, she is the favorite of most of the men in the crowd, and there is a glandular lustiness in the applause she gets from them. Kike's routine is graceful and athletic, but is done to a kind of stripper-disco piece of music that seems wrong for her. Laura Combes poses to a wonderful piece of music and practically every woman backstage crowds into the wings to watch her arrogant, muscular, fist-clenching routine. But the routine that brings down the house is done to the song "Endless Love" by a slender, pretty black girl—a Philadelphia native named Karen Wainright whose husband, also a bodybuilder, had been shot and killed earlier in the week.

After Ron Teufel and Franco Columbu guest-pose, it is announced that there will be a poseoff among the

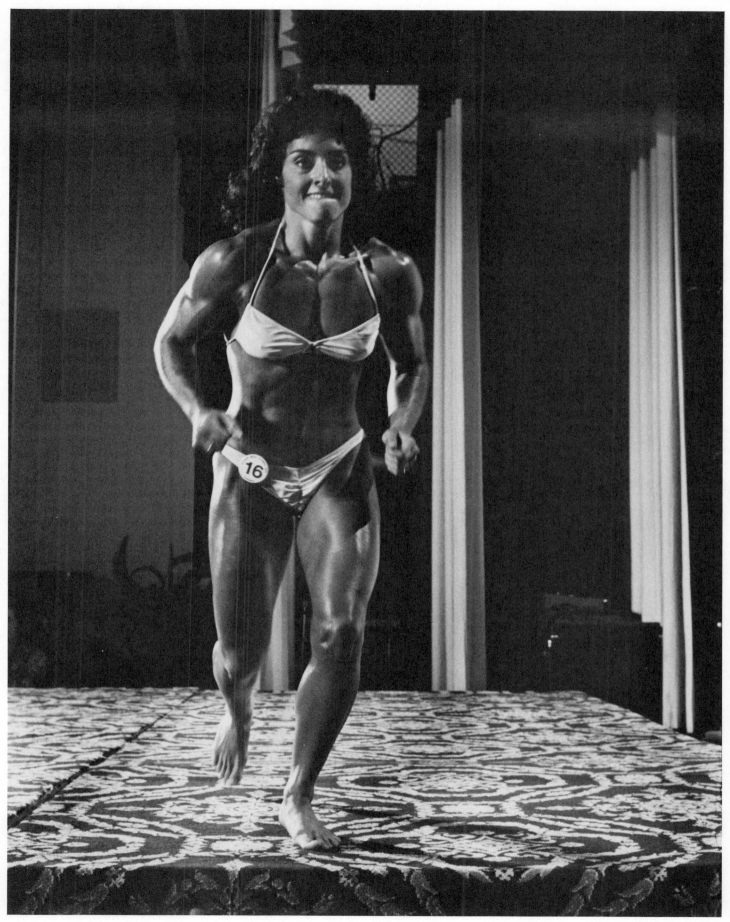

Laura Combes

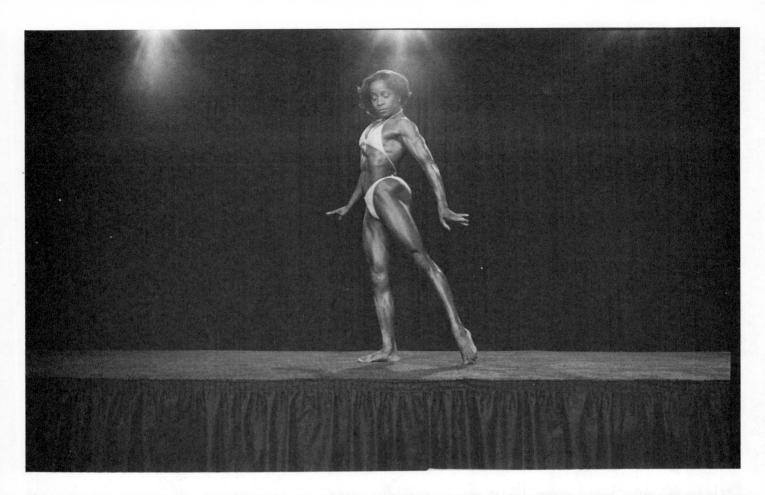

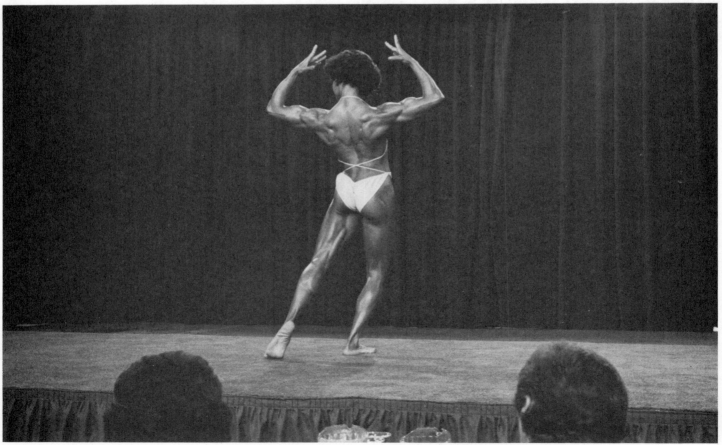

Carla Dunlap, performing

"When I won the Miss Olympia last year I thought, I know what I have to do for next year—I know exactly what I have to do. I still have the same balance and proportions and I've got the cuts, now I'm going to really point out to the world what bodybuilding is: build your body to enhance the feminine physique. And this is what I dedicated this whole year to . . . . I gained eight pounds."
—Rachel McLish

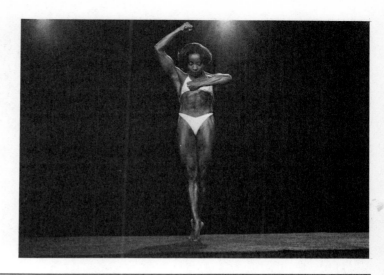

six finalists in which the judges can award further points, thereby possibly altering slightly the results of the afternoon's prejudging at which those six finalists were chosen and ranked. With "Celebration" playing and the crowd going crazy, Georgia Miller Fudge, Lynn Conkwright, Rachel McLish, Corinne Machado-Ching, Candy Csencsits and Kike Elomaa take the stage and simultaneously begin hitting poses. This is the peak moment in male bodybuilding shows—the time when whatever it is that is fascinating about competing physiques becomes most vivid, and the chaos of shifting curves and straight lines of muscle on the stage takes on an immediacy, a combative energy, that somehow clarifies and shapes it. None of that happens with the women. A posedown among women bodybuilders looks sort of like a chorus line run amok. But with the irresistible beat of "Celebration" behind it and a number of truly stunning bodies involved, this one gets the audience behind it anyway, and for a few moments turns into something vital. In the heat of it some inflamed man at a table near the stage keeps screaming a question to Rachel McLish. Finally, in a shift between poses, she looks down toward her bare stomach, at the object of his curiosity. "It's a *birthmark,*" she shouts to him over the music.

If the poseoff is a disappointment, what follows is a disgrace, symbolically telling if not necessarily characteristic of women's bodybuilding at this stage in its development. It and a fistfight that occurs later that night between two women, one of them a bodybuilder, were all anyone was talking about the next day at the Philadelphia Sheraton, and that too seemed symbolic. When the poseoff finalists were announced after the prejudging, a lot of people out front and backstage had wondered what had happened to Laura Combes, including Laura herself. Now everyone finds out when the places are announced after the posedown.

Oscar State stands in front of the mike and clears his throat. Sixth place, he says, goes to Candy Csencsits.

Candy comes on stage beaming to the applause and takes her trophy. Fifth place: Georgia Miller Fudge. Still a little teary, Georgia walks out and accepts her trophy. And fourth place, says Oscar, with a cash prize of three thousand dollars, goes to . . . Laura Combes! If everyone else in the entire ballroom is confused, Laura isn't. Not called out for the posedown, she had known all along she belonged in it. Bouncing onto the stage from out front somewhere, she tears off the warmup suit covering her bikini and begins hitting poses for the befuddled but wildly cheering audience, while Corinne Machado-Ching, the object of Oscar's apparent mistake, stands in the wings with the other three contestants for only three places left, trying bravely to smile.

The next morning Roger Schwab, one of the judges, told me that when he heard Oscar announce the six finalists for the posedown he had simply thrown his pencil up in the air. Roger had Laura either first or second on his card and he knew that she couldn't have possibly placed lower than sixth. Corinne Machado-Ching had actually placed seventh. When Oscar State had gotten to fourth place in the poseoff announcement, he must have somehow read down a few lines below and called out Corinne's name instead of Laura's. He had kept the toting-up of scores completely to himself, had refused to let anyone else, even Doris, the other head judge, have a look at the totals, and the grumble that next morning was that it wasn't the first mistake the old British codger had made, and it wouldn't be the last. If so, this particular mistake denied Laura Combes extra points in the poseoff and therefore might have cost her third place, which was won by Lynn Conkwright, or even, Laura believed, second or first.

Rachel McLish and Kike Elomaa stand side by side in the wings. Laura has had her avenging flurry of poses and has accepted her trophy. Lynn Conkwright has accepted hers, looking cheery and fresh as a summer morning. Rachel and Kike wait for the next announce-

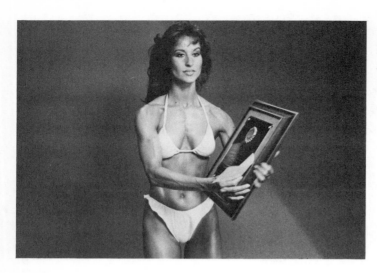

"Last year I got calls from people who wanted me to wrestle men for seven thousand dollars. I said are you kidding me? I'm not going to make a sideshow out of bodybuilding."
—Rachel McLish

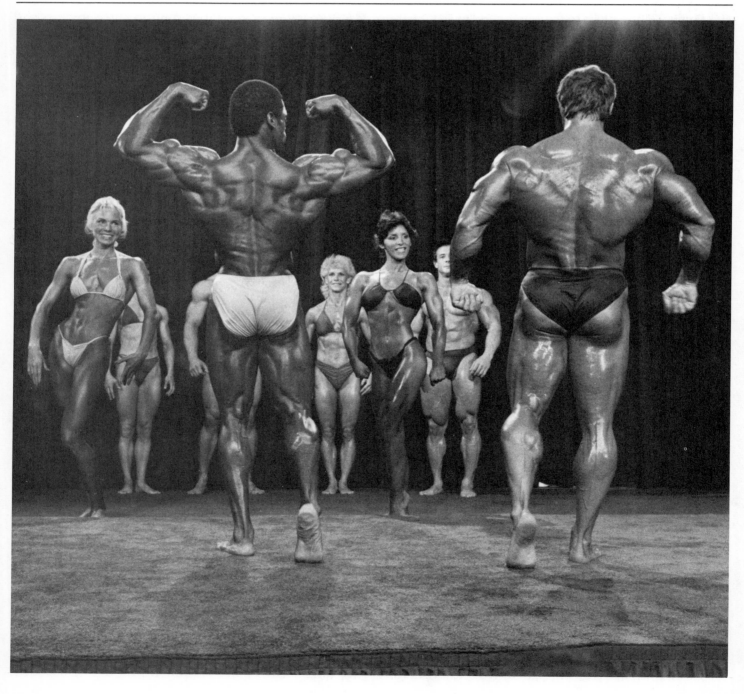

ment, two pretty women with strong legs and no fat, one more marketable than the other, both ambitious and bright and hard-working, and hopeful that their bodies can make them rich and famous in the odd, unsettled sport of women's bodybuilding. Rachel's head is bent; her eyes are closed and there is a prayerful expression on her face. Kike looks expectant, eager to hear what she knows is coming.

"Second place," says Oscar State, "with a cash prize of six thousand dollars, goes to Rachel McLish."

The next morning Rachel McLish was angry and confused. "At first," she said, "I thought Kike's got a nice physique. I naturally thought mine was better because I scrutinize females—I've been a body watcher from way back. I felt I had better lines and I was the defending champion and the ideal, and I had everything going for me. And here the defending champion is so much more *improved,* I mean I look so much better than last year. I had everything going for me and I felt so confident; I thought for sure I was going to win and it was tight up until the third round and I naturally had more experience in posing and in being in front of an audience, and of course the audience response was really great and everything. Then they had the poseoff. . . . I did my best. I wasn't looking over my shoulder. I was just doing my thing. I couldn't concern myself with who was standing next to me, and when they announced the winner I thought well I've got to hand it to this girl. She must have really done great."

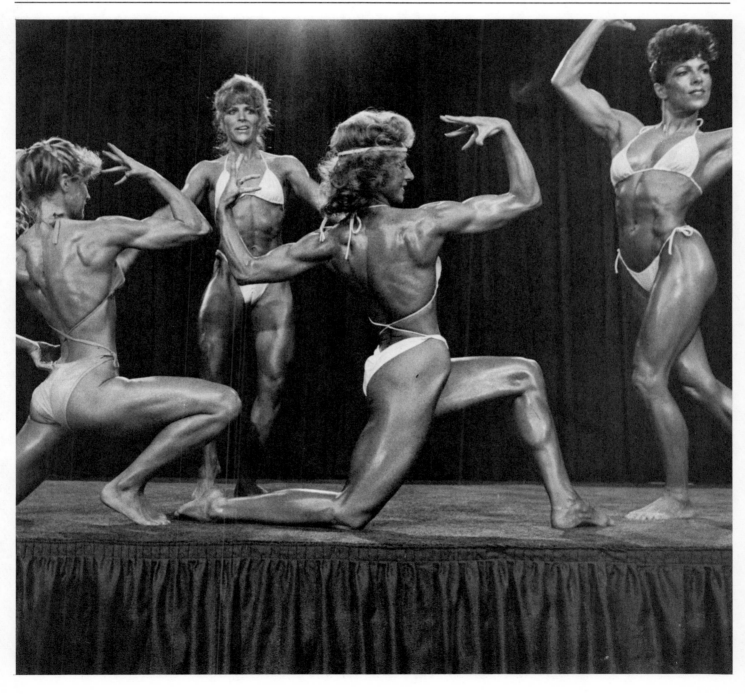

When asked what her plans were, Rachel said she wasn't going to enter any more contests for a while. "I'm going to wait until they get set criteria for judging," she said. "Until the judging standards are set, I won't stand on the stage anymore."

Corinne Machado-Ching was also, and understandably, angry and confused; and so was Laura Combes, who had no way of knowing whether the final results were an endorsement of her sort of development or not. And so were Kike and Kimmo Elomaa, who were learning that morning that at least part of what the bodybuilding writer had told me the day before was true. Despite Kike's triumph, riches and fame were no closer at hand. Half of her ten-thousand-dollar first place prize money, said Kimmo, would go to Finnish

customs. They were hanging around the hotel waiting for someone to offer her an endorsement contract or something, but so far no one had. They had had an appointment with a magazine publisher, but he hadn't showed.

"I think that everyone has tried to avoid us," said Kimmo. "I don't know why, but I think that Americans want to keep the winning to themselves. Now because Kike is the first foreign woman who has ever won any American prize, I think it is very hard for them to realize that."

A lovely, poised, hard-to-market foreign woman had won it, but the real upshot of the 1981 Professional Women's Bodybuilding Championships was anger and confusion among the contestants, both winners and

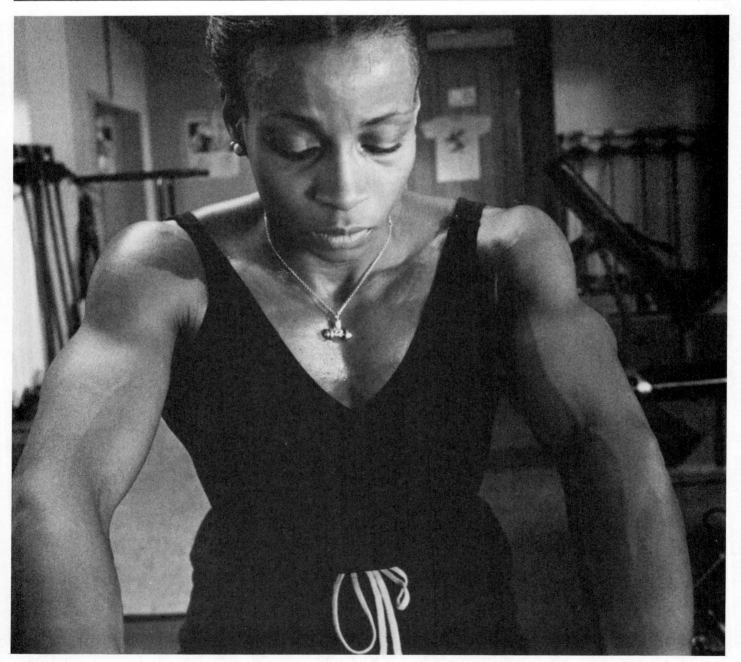

Carla Dunlap

losers, a fistfight over a man between two women involved in the competition, a disastrous mistake committed in the tabulation of the contest results, and a further extension of the dispute over what the judges should be judging in the first place. The day after the contest at the Philadelphia Sheraton felt like a hangover. There were no more deal makers hustling the suites and lobby, and it might well have seemed to even the most optimistic observer that the sport of women's bodybuilding had at least as far to go as it did from this same place one year before. The big question that year had been how far *can* it go; this year, the day after the contest, the questions seemed to be: Can it go at all, and if so who is going to pay the freight?

Now, in 1984, those are still the questions.

"For three years I've argued that there are two types of women and that the solution would be two types of contests. Except for one Florida promoter, I've met nothing but opposition, yet this is where the controversy lies. How many men with narrow shoulders and wide hips win the men's contests?"
—Doris Barrilleaux

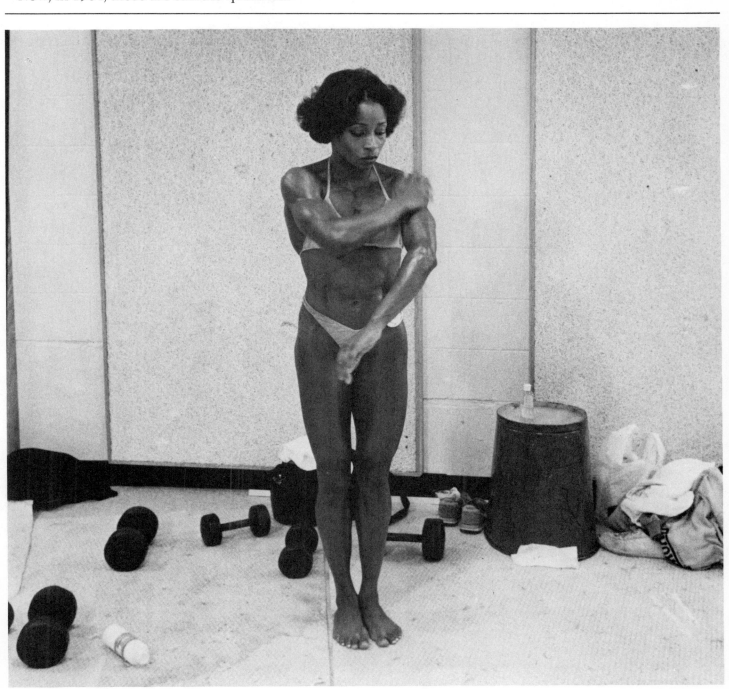

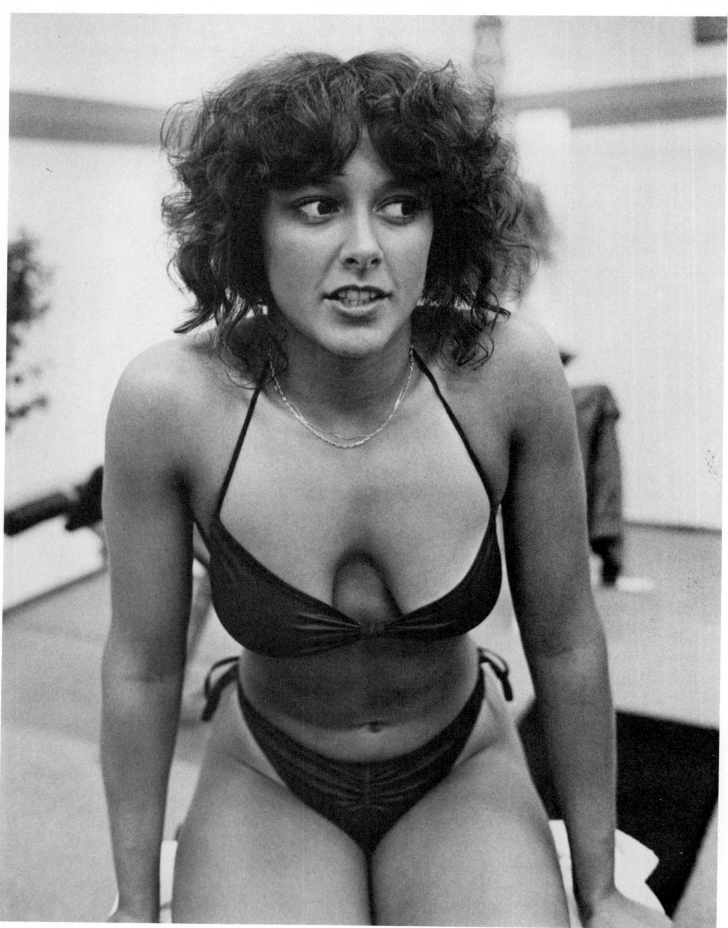

DeeDee Antonelli, Stone's Gym, 1981

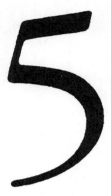

The short-class women are standing in a line along a stairway leading up to the stage of the Berkeley Performance Center in Boston, Massachusetts, waiting to go on for the prejudging of the 1981 Miss Northeast Contest. They are all oiled up, nervous and illuminated by red bulbs, so that their bare, oily, nervous skin gives off a pink glow. Most of them use the steps to get in a few last-minute calf-raises.

"Bodybuilding gives you ulcers, but who cares?" says one woman. Another one chuckles wryly.

"I've got some lipstick if anybody wants any," says another.

"Gloss or color?"

At the bottom of the stairs a few of the women are talking about Kike Elomaa.

"I love her legs."

"God, is she in the bucks."

"She's won thirty-five thousand *dollars*. She's European champ, and then, you know, the Olympia. She's *loaded*."

In the auditorium there are over three hundred people, a lot for the prejudging of a regional show with no big names entered in it. Audiences at the big national female bodybuilding competitions tend to be well dressed, more or less evenly divided between men and women, reserved, kind in their responses, and aesthetically as unsure of themselves as everybody else in the sport (a high energy, such as Auby Paulick's, is the only quality in a competitor sure to arouse them). They seem self-conscious, those audiences—on their good behavior and tentative about what they are watching—and you rarely find among them in any numbers the noisy, opinionated super-fan types who have always given the male competitions much of their color and excitement.

The audience here at the Miss Northeast is mostly male and young. There are a lot of male bodybuilders in it (there was a Mr. Northeast going on that day too), and a lot of family of both the men and women competitors. It is a loud, responsive, happy crowd, here to

see what it can see and hoping to see something special. A partisan segment of it comes from the area around Hanover, Massachusetts, southeast of Boston, and those people are here because Lenny Archambault has brought some of his girls to compete. Lenny is a good northeastern bodybuilder who has been around for a long time and has had over the years some top finishes in a few national contests. He is deservedly known as a first-rate poser, and for the past few months he has been running a posing class for women at a place called Stone's Gym in Hanover. He also trains some of the women to whom he gives posing lessons, and he has brought four of them here today for their first competition.

The short class comes on, and there is not much in it. As with male bodybuilding, when the posing and the physiques are less than very good, the showing off of nearly naked, oily bodies can be embarrassing, depressing or silly. Or even all three, as is the case with a stoned-looking girl with a flower in her hair who whirls her undeveloped self around in slow pirouettes with neither grace nor design, and at one point actually lies down on the stage in such an apparent stupor that there is a real question as to whether or not she will get back up. One woman named Chris saves the class with some muscle and a dignified routine, posing with her legs arranged at pretty angles and a calm, happy expression on her face. The tall class is better overall, and in it are two women, both students of Lenny's, who are great to look at. One of them, DeeDee Antonelli, has clearly just begun to train. She has a lovely, feminine body which is starting to tighten up around the edges, and a somber, beautiful face. The other has terrific presence, a bright, pretty, energetic face, and a physique which is not too far from being as good as any in the sport. She is the easy class of the competition, the sort of star in the rough you go to regional contests hoping to see, and the crowd loves her. Her name, according to the program, is Cindy Hardee.

Between the compulsory and free-posing segments

of the prejudging I go backstage with two of my children to look up Lenny Archambault. He says he is running his posing classes on a weekly basis and invites me down to Stone's Gym to watch one of them. Cindy Hardee is standing nearby hamming it up in a mirror for a couple of appreciative male bodybuilders. She directs a pose at me into the mirror to get my attention, her face literally popping with energy.

"You should come down and watch us train," she says.

I say that I'd like to, and tell her I hope she wins the contest. I ask her how long she has been training.

Only four weeks, she says.

Impressed, I ask her what kind of routine she is on. We have an audience now. Cindy looks back into the mirror and hits a chest shot, her hands on her hips. She grins at herself.

"Sex," she says. "Sex really cuts you up."

George Butler and I finally went down to Stone's Gym together in January 1982. We arrived around two in the afternoon and were met by Lenny and by Bruce and Janet Stone, the owners. The Stones are a couple of various parts. She is a commodities broker and a published novelist. Together they own a successful beef importing business and a gym equipment manufacturing company in addition to the gym, which is one of the best I've been in—a huge place with good Stone workout equipment, lots of natural light, and the bouncy, juiced-up, energetic feeling of all good gyms.

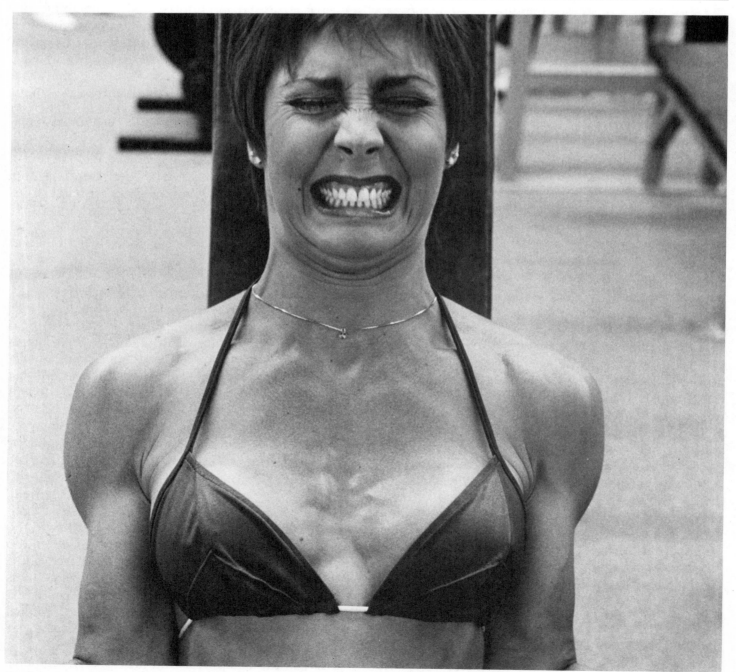

Cindy Hardee

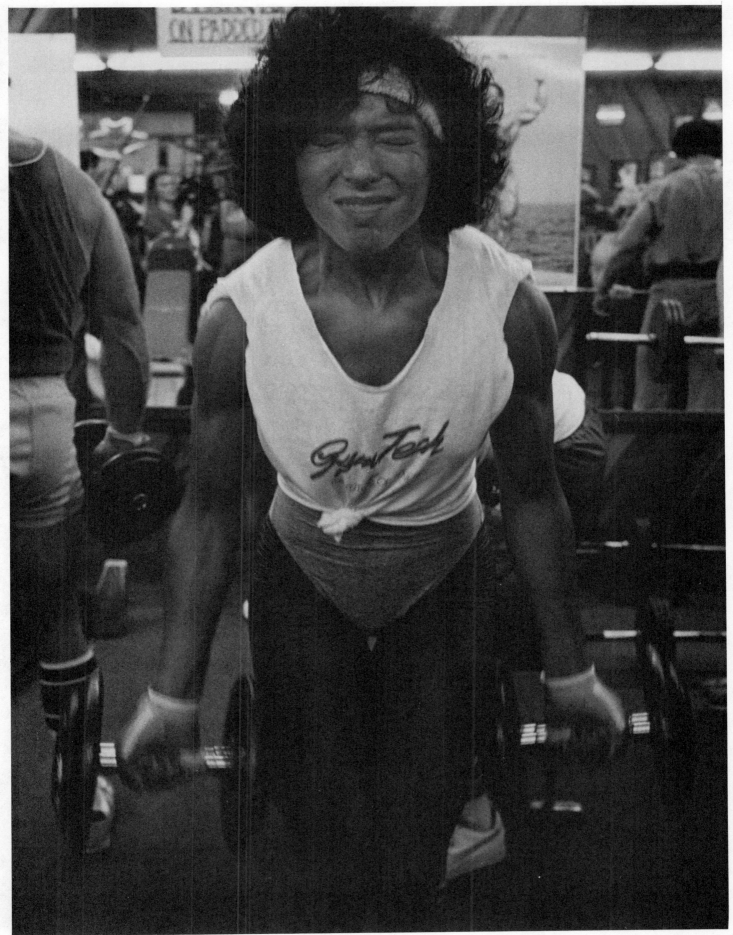

Lydia Cheng

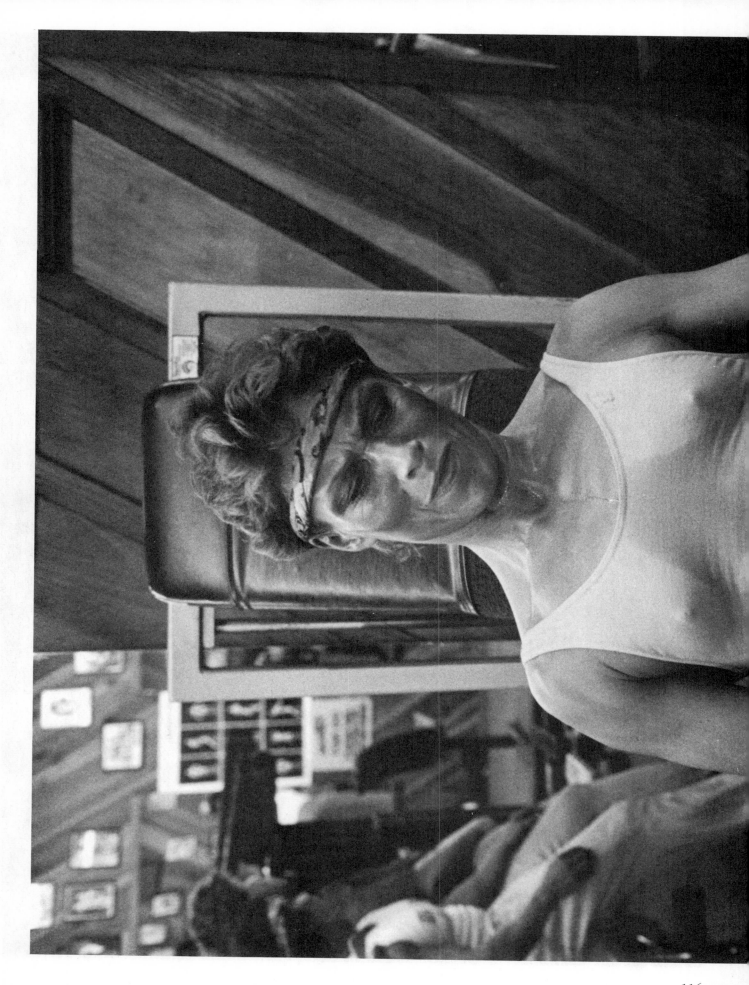

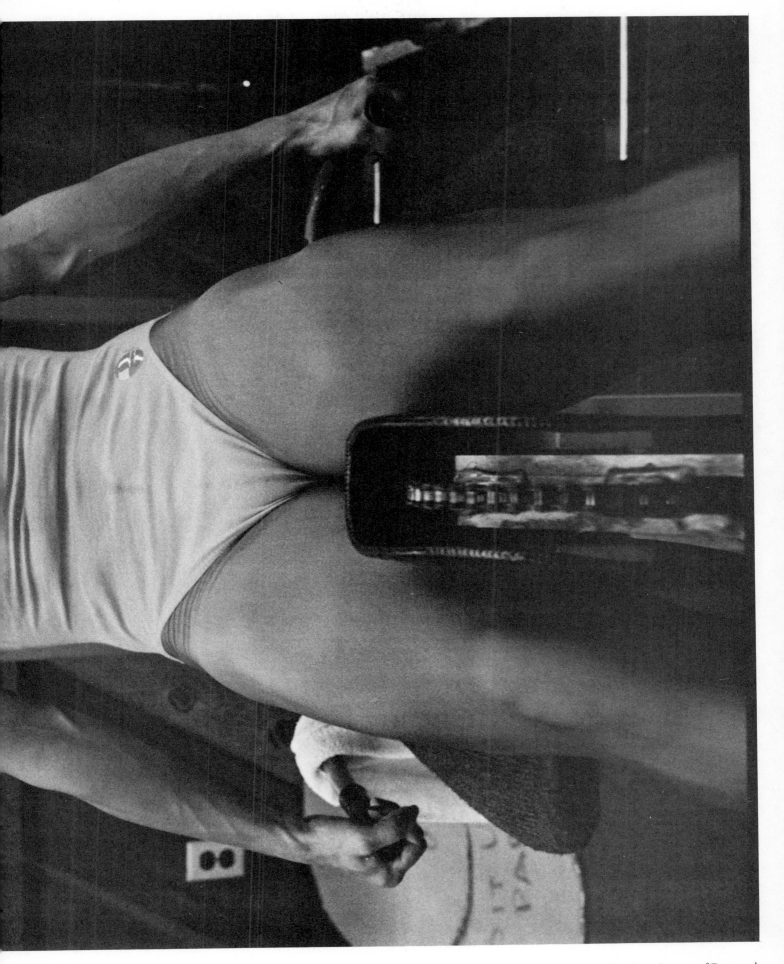

Lisa Frost Larsen of Denmark

It is not one of the all-women bodybuilding gyms which are sprouting up around the country, like Spunky's outside Detroit and Muscles in Miami and Mid-City in Manhattan; it is coed, and both the men and the women I talked to there said they liked training together.

"Third Rate Romance" was playing on the stereo, there were eight or nine male bodybuilders using the facilities, and seven of Lenny's women bodybuilders were standing around, looking good, ready for posing class. Of the seven, Cindy and DeeDee were the farthest along in their training, and they were clearly Lenny's favorites. The women stripped down to their posing suits and stood together on a big dais set up before a mirror in one of the gym's spare rooms, oiling each other, joking and getting psyched. Cindy Hardee had been training hard since I saw her at the Miss Northeast in September, and her body was both more defined and rounder. DeeDee's body was also further along, and just then flushed with niacin she had taken to redden her skin. Other women were mixing iodine with baby oil to give themselves the semblance of a tan in the middle of this New England winter. Except for Cindy and DeeDee none of them looked like bodybuilders, though all but two had competed at it and all of them trained regularly.

Lenny, who wore a T-shirt over his bulging upper body proclaiming him "The Wizard of Posing," started in with a girl who had never posed before and showed her how to stand for the relaxed poses. The other

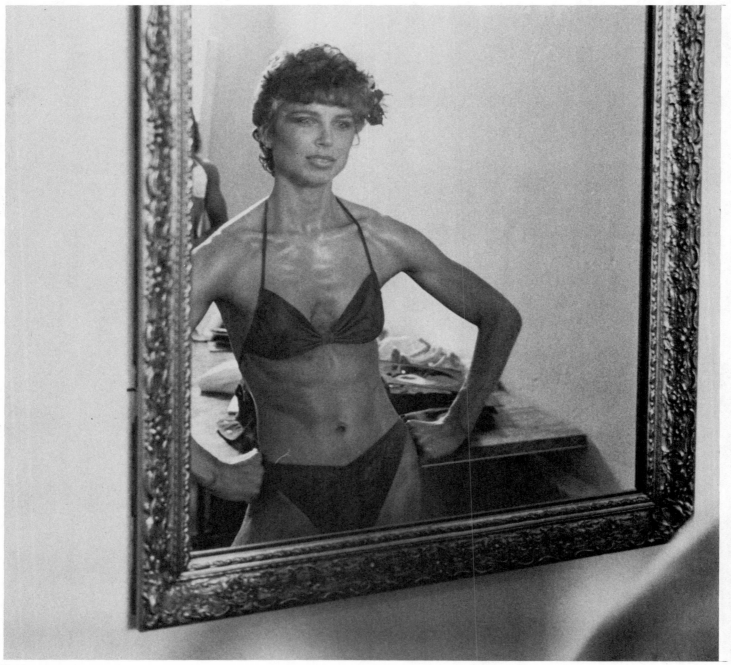

Barbara Lamb

118

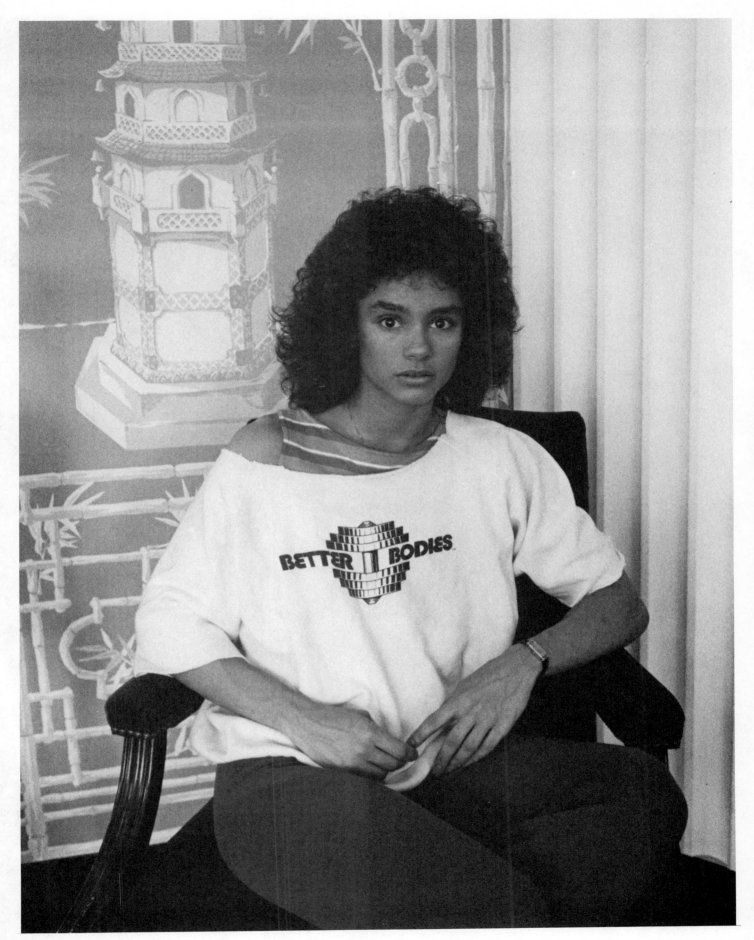

Gladys Portugues

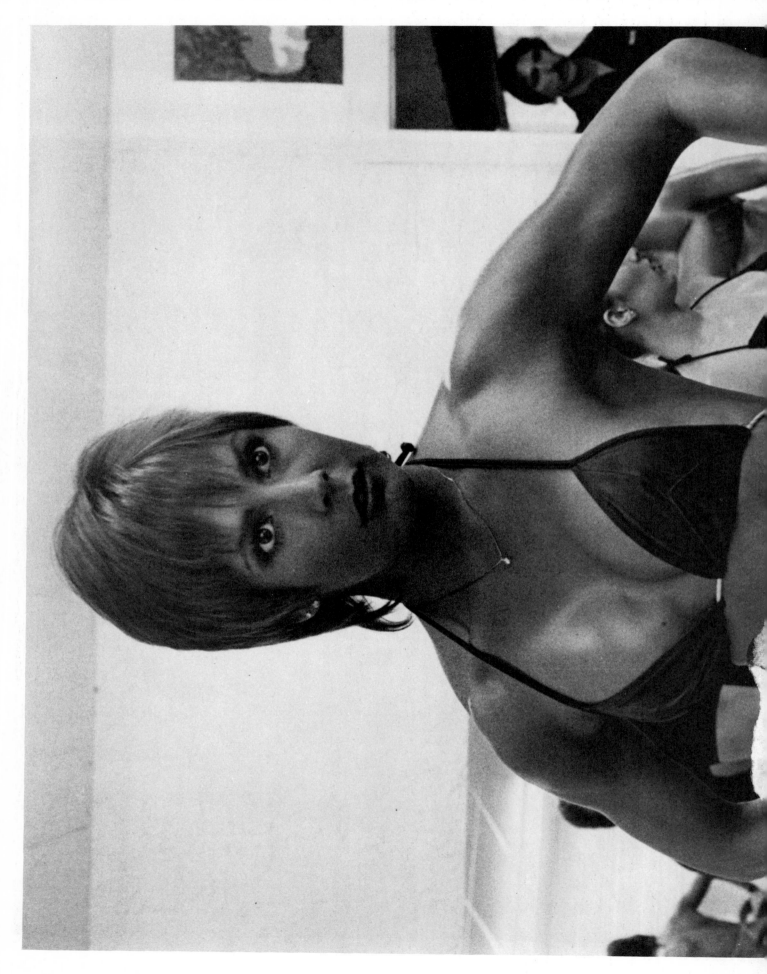

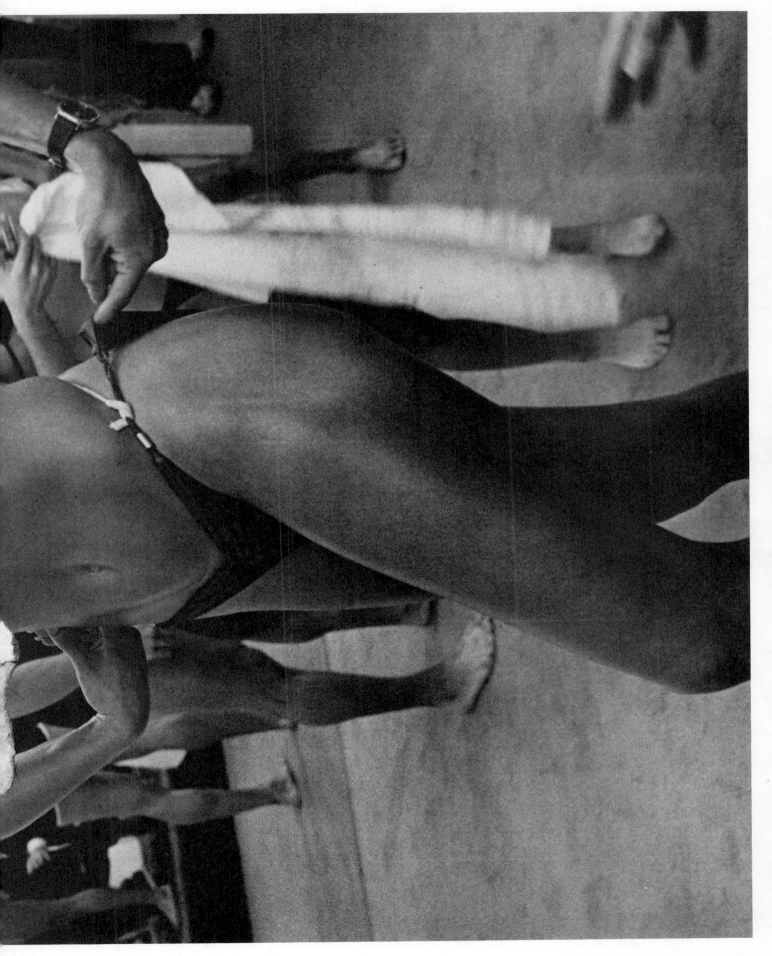

Cindy Hardee, Stone's Gym, 1982

"I love the morning. I'm a morning person. I love sunrises. I'm very aesthetic. I love nature. I go with Steve and we go hunting every week. I love fast cars. I want to talk about food. Food is definitely next to sex in my book. For many years that's all I had, food."
—Cindy Hardee

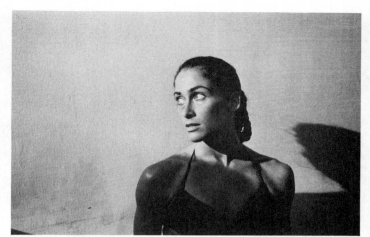

Melinda Perper

women grouped together in front of the dais, saying, "Good," and "Oh, great," as The Wizard led the woman through the moves and showed her how to stand sideways to look four inches taller.

"Your shoulders are always square," he said, adjusting her body with his hands. "In other words you want to look like you're straight all the time, but you're not, because you want your waist to look tiny. When you make your waist look tiny, it makes you look taller. It makes you look broader in the shoulders. There you have your symmetry. Now turn again. Turn to the side. That's what I want. I want you to exaggerate first, and then we'll straighten it out from there. That's good. Bend this leg out. More. Now the arch in the back is very important. Very important. See, the smaller the ribcage, the smaller the waist. Now. How tall are you, five foot two? And you look a whole lot taller. Now go back to your normal way and look. It doesn't show anything. Turn your head to the side, either side. Go right around. Turn again. Shoulders back. Very good. Now step down and I want Denise to go through this. The same thing."

He told Denise that he wanted her to "open up. I want you to blossom. Keep your arms straight down. All I want you to do here is widen your back, 'cause you have a good back. There it is. Now don't bend this knee quite so much. Lean. Straighten this leg right out. This one. There, straighten it right out. Arch your back. Okay, good . . ."

The other women encouraged each poser in turn. "Feminine hands, baby," said Cindy Hardee, juking to the music on the stereo. "Keep them feminine." And, "Straighten your leg, honey."

Lenny chose Cindy for a free-posing demonstration, and she went through it perfectly, grinning like crazy and blowing on her bangs. Then DeeDee posed, with nice, serious moves, her lovely, dark, Florentine face studious. Lenny ended the session with himself and Cindy in a double-posing routine. They planned to compete together in the couples' competition in Atlan-

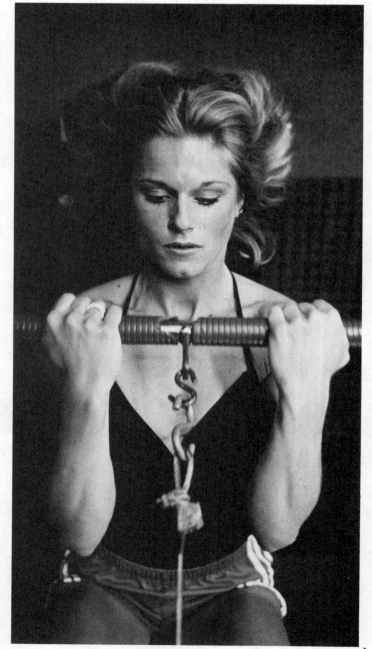

Terri Le Cicero

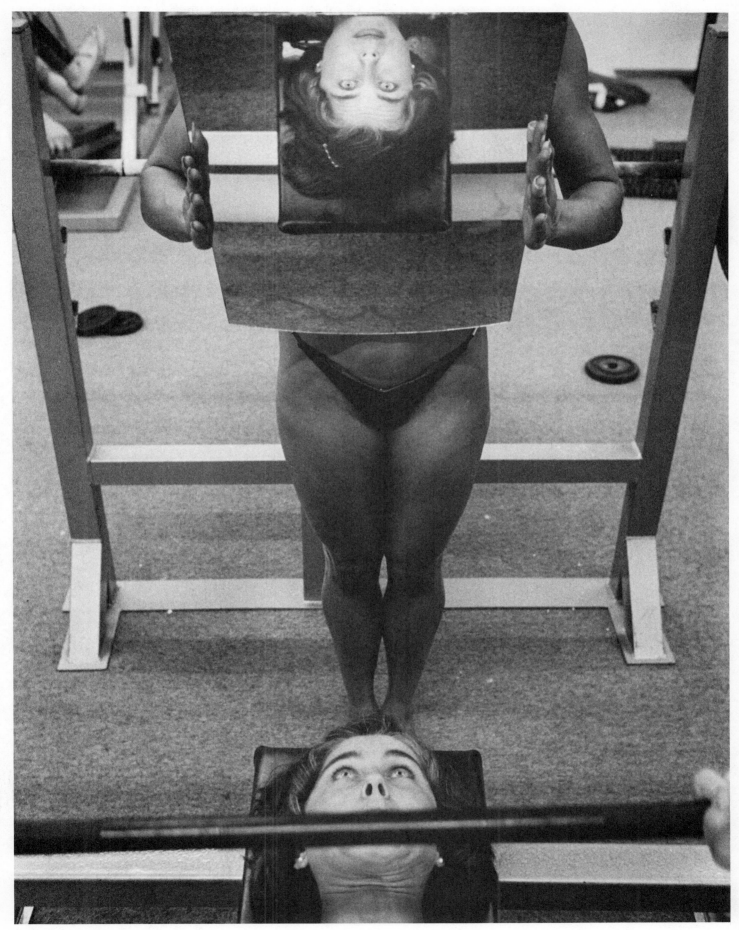

Lenny's training secret

123

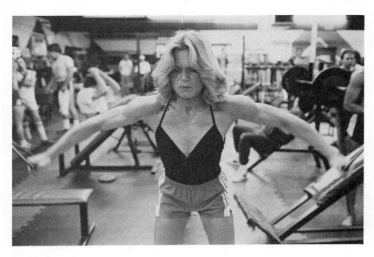

tic City the following spring and were still working out the routine.

"Now we're gonna go down, Cyn," Lenny said, sweeping Cindy into one of the melodramatic, ballroom-dance-like movements of couples posing. "Down we go. Look up. And now we're gonna come up. Go 'round. Go 'round again. I like that. Now we're gonna . . . Where do you want to go from here?" Cindy suggested a move. "No," said the Wizard. "Keep going here. On my knee and up. That's nice. Now when we come up we're gonna turn like this. Now I want you to go down on my knee on this side. You follow me? Keep your hands open. Now we're gonna come up and turn right around. Up you go, and open it up to finish. There . . . that's not bad."

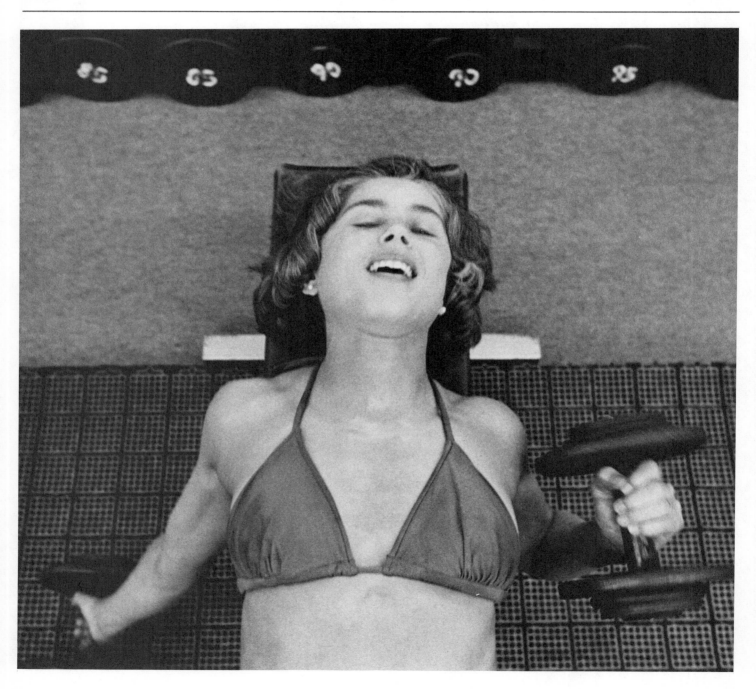

Lenny's women pay him twenty-five dollars apiece for a lesson, and it takes eight to ten lessons before a competitor is considered stage ready. All of the women there seemed to feel they were getting their money's worth whether they ever won a contest or not, and there was no question, watching the class, that The Wizard brought some magic to what he did, managing to make even the most awkward of the women look and feel graceful on the dais.

When I asked him about his occupation he said, "I teach women how to have femininity. I pull the elegance out of them and make them understand what posing is all about. If you come onstage showing that you're in control of yourself, you give people goose pimples right up and down their backs. They get all

"When you're teaching a woman how to pose you're touching her and showing her different movements and you have to stay professional. If you start thinking about how sexy she looks and how she stimulates you, then you're in trouble."
—Lenny Archambault

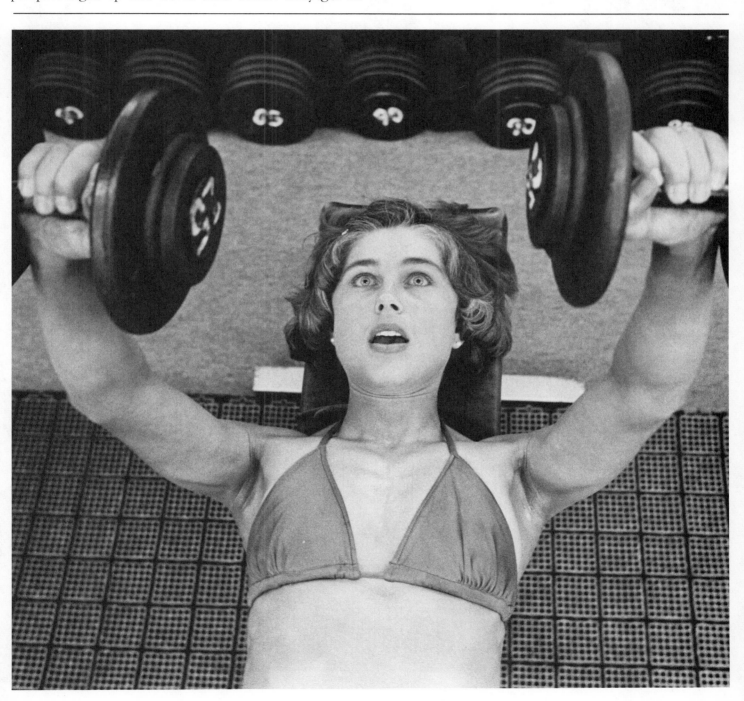

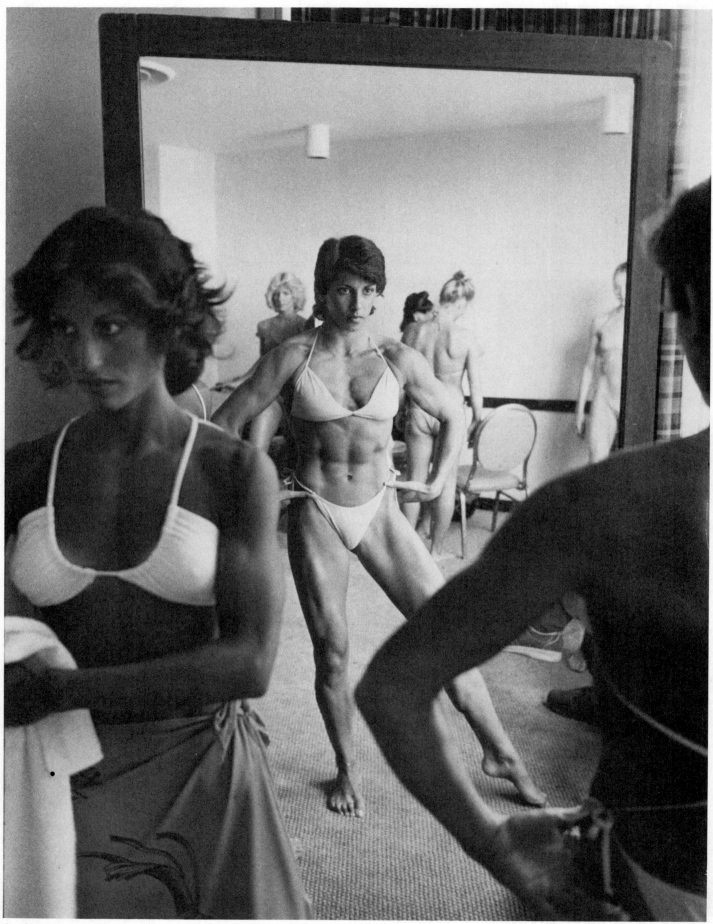

Check-posing

excited because half of the people in that audience want to be onstage too, but they don't dare. If they see somebody who isn't together, they get nervous for that person and it bothers them. But when they see somebody up there who has it together—wow! They're in *awe*. That's what you try to do. You try to teach them how to bring what they have across. I tell my women to begin with that there's nobody onstage as good as they are. So who's gonna beat them? Because nobody can pose as good as my women. I know this. This gives them confidence because they feel that I'm behind them. That's all they have to know, is that I'm there. I'm there when they're onstage. I'm in the audience. I'm backstage with them. And I don't just cater to one woman, I cater to all the women I have trained. I treat

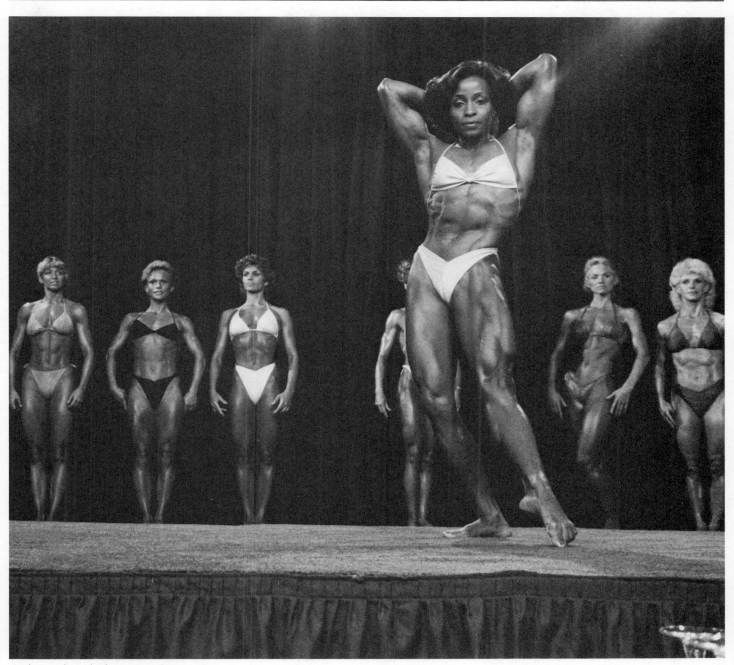

Carla Dunlap, ab shot, prejudging

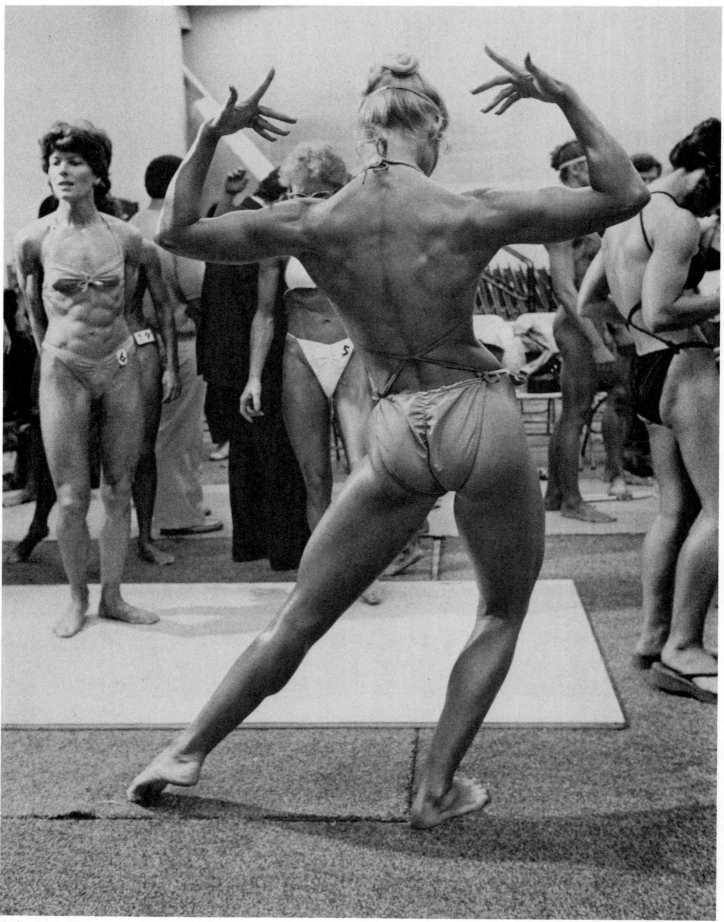

Shelly Gruwell

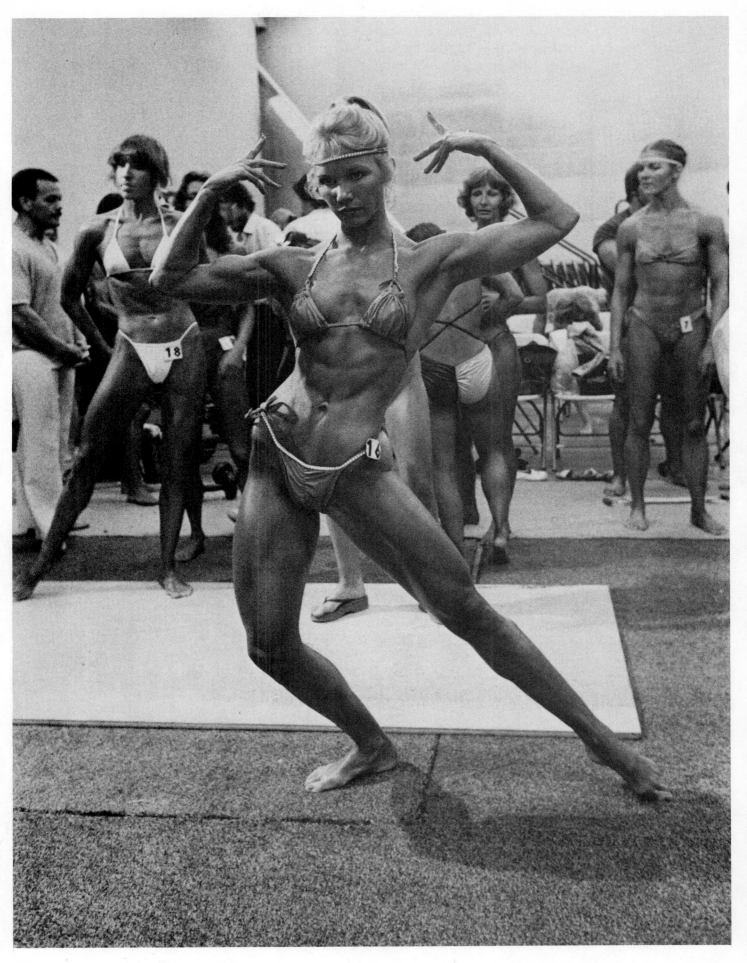

'em equal and this is why I think they perform so well. That's why I am The Wizard of Posing. They relax with me because I get into their minds. I relax with them. I don't try to be Mr. Macho Man and say I'm the king here and you're a little girl and I'm gonna show you what you're gonna do. I don't do that. I treat them equal to me."

After the class, Lenny took his women into the gym to train. As a rule women bodybuilders do not train with the same pain-blind ferocity that the men do. Most good male bodybuilders love pain. "No pain, no gain," is the motto of their workouts. And the best of them stalk around a gym looking at the dumbbells and bars like linebackers look at wide receivers, anticipating with relish their collisions with them and the resultant pain. Most of the women seem almost to toy with the weights, and rarely will carry a set out to the point where the last few reps are done through any real pain. Their workouts are delicate and precise, prim in comparison to those of male bodybuilders and, judging by the ones I have seen, not as much fun. Because women have a higher percentage of fat than men do, women bodybuilders' workouts usually include a lot of fat-burning high-rep lightweight exercises. This is particularly true of the gymnast–ballet dancer body types like Lynn Conkwright, who for her midsection does three sets of three hundred sit-ups, three sets of one hundred trunk twists, and three sets of one hundred side bends, fifty repetitions of leg thrusts for her legs, and rarely fewer than twenty repetitions of any exer-

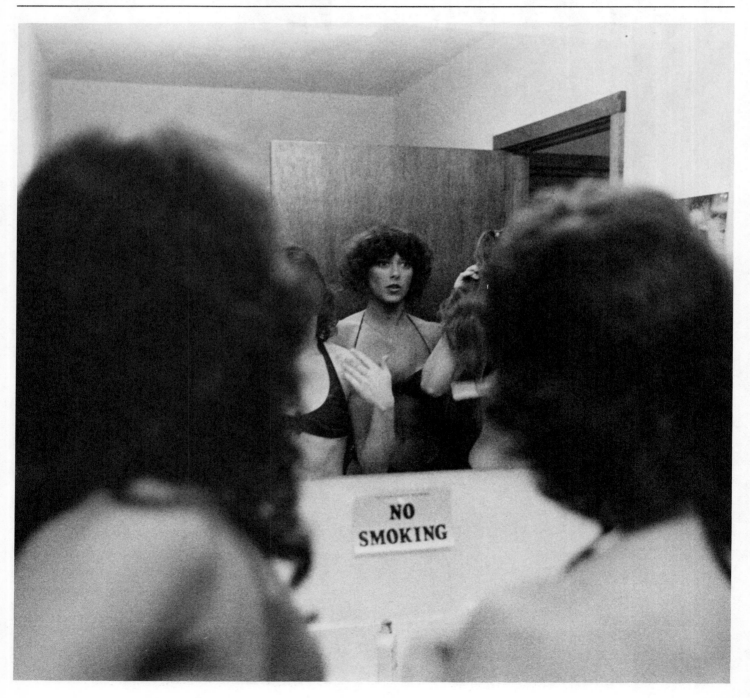

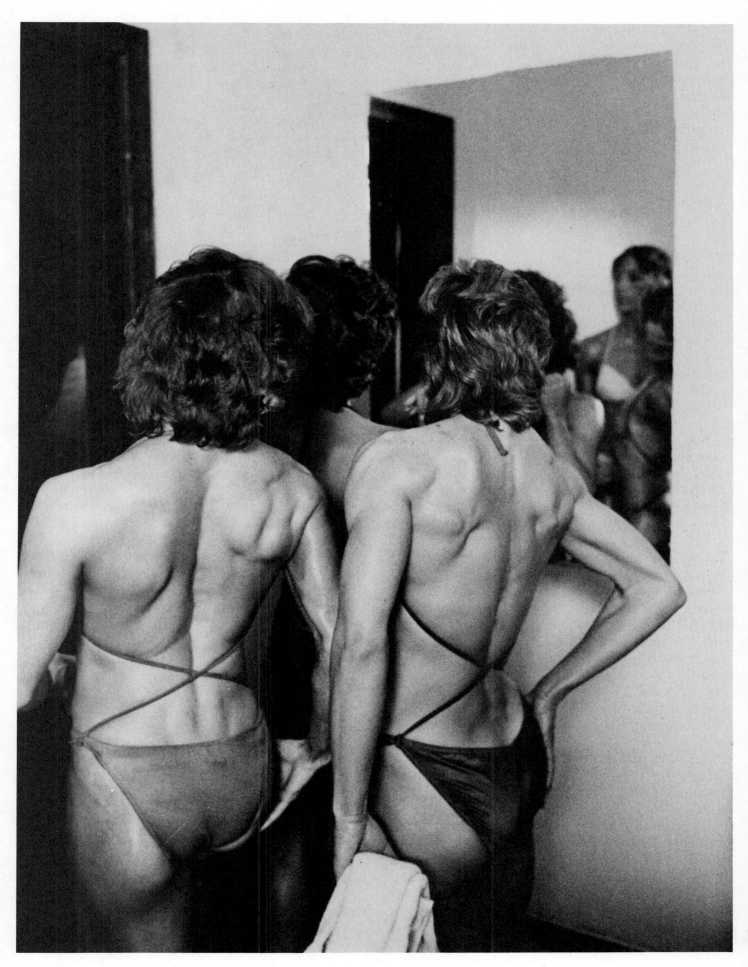

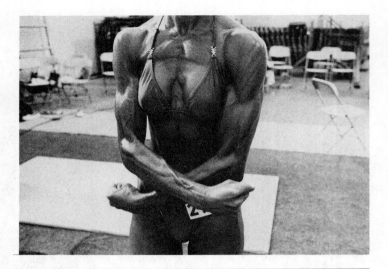

cise for her upper body. (By contrast, Auby Paulick—who trains for heavier, rounder muscles, and is sometimes criticized for them as looking too masculine—does between eight and ten reps for most exercises, using, for the most part, much heavier weights than Lynn uses, in a routine that is similar to a male bodybuilder's.)

Cindy Hardee, DeeDee Antonelli and the others dabbled with the weights that day at Stone's Gym after the posing class, more out of convenience for George Butler's camera than for real training. Lenny, their trainer, had come up with a new technique: for those exercises in which they could not see themselves in the gym's wall mirrors, he would hold a smaller mirror in front of the part of the body being exercised and tilt the reflection so that they could see it. It increased their concentration, said The Wizard, and he asked me not to tell anyone on the West Coast about it.

If watching women bodybuilders pose and compete is not generally sexually stimulating, watching them train can be. They do not pump up as noticeably or quickly as men do, and they don't train with the same sort of abandon and lust, but they flush and they sweat and they moan, and their bodies become ripely colored and subtly swollen with the exercises. Doing inclined curls and flyes, both Cindy and DeeDee looked a little orgasmic, with things flashing in their fine chests.

When they were finished I asked Cindy to come and stand in front of me, relaxed, so that I could study her, as you might a piece of sculpture. Here is the report: She has a thin neck and good round trapezius muscles connecting her neck to her wide shoulders; narrow, well-defined lats that drop sharply to her small ribcage and waist; and high, taut, generous breasts. Her arms are smoothly muscled and long, her hips narrow, her thighs rounded and strong-looking; her knees and ankles are small, and her calves perfect heart shapes between them. From the back you notice the vertical lines: the steep slant from her shoulders to her waist,

the lovely, womanly bell-curve of buttocks and the athlete's outward flaring of the thighs. From the side there is the wonderful reversed S-shape of a woman's profile, in this case sharper and more precisely balanced than usual, and again the muscular push of the thigh line.

About some of the bodies in female bodybuilding—some of the bodies pictured in this book—it must be admitted there is an existential strangeness. A quantitative extension of anything we are accustomed to looking at becomes after a certain point a qualitatively new thing, often disturbingly new. Most of us, male or female, can appreciate a female body viscerally and visually *as* a female body only up to a certain point of modification; beyond that point, modification registers as distortion and we feel that we are looking at something disturbingly *other than* the original thing. This may be particularly true of the female body, loaded as it is with visual biological symbolism. Strip a woman's body of its breasts and hips, of all its nurturing curves, and replace it with enough stringy, sinewy muscle, and a lot of people will simply not know what to make of what you have left. They may say it looks like a man; what they really mean is that, in no longer looking like a woman, it has become visually, existentially, strange: unknowable.

The best of the present female bodybuilders do not look distorted or strange—they simply look modified. (The ultimate woman bodybuilder, the one who will finally put the art and sport together, will look neither modified nor distorted; hers will be at the same time a perfectly natural and a brand-new version of the female body.) Sometimes their modifications are beautiful, often without specific reference to the amount of muscle they entail. As with everything that strikes the eye, a certain amount of gratuitous grace is involved in bodybuilding. Cindy Hardee's modifications are small but the results are beautiful; her body is beautifully made, provocative and stirring, and though it has muscles, more than some well-developed teenaged boys have, no one in his or her right mind could accuse it

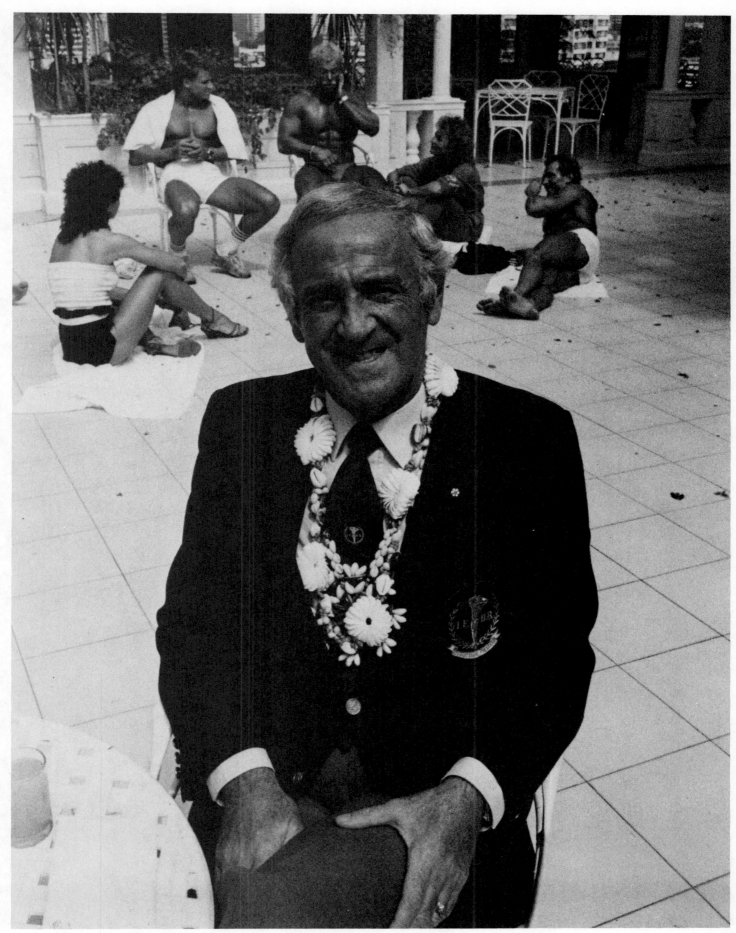

Ben Weider, female bodybuilding aesthete

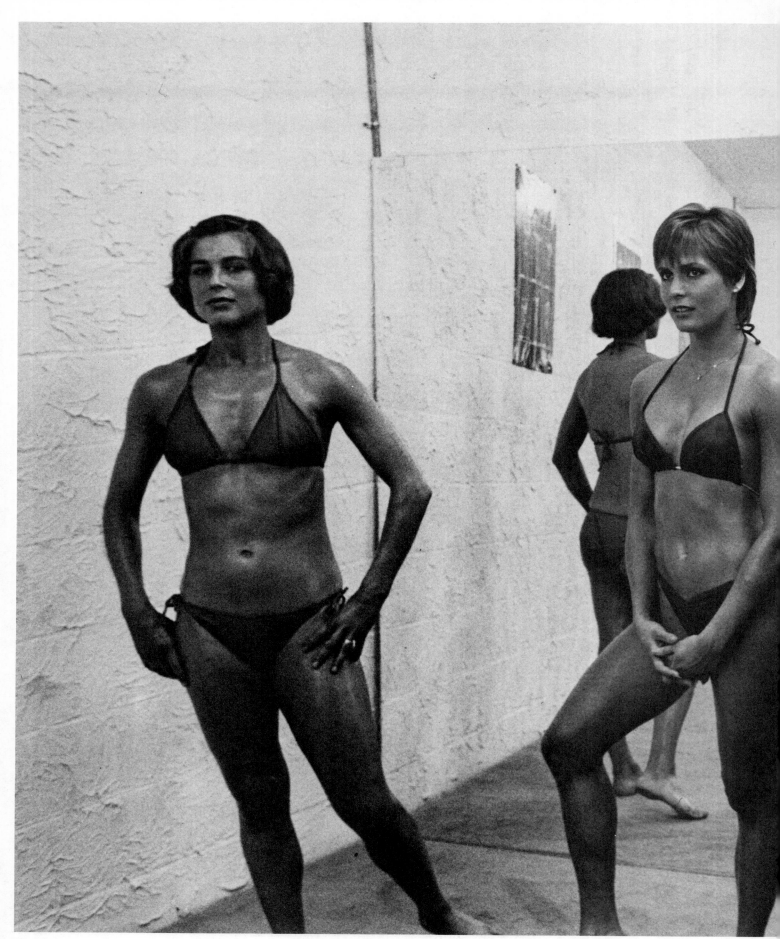

Stone's Gym

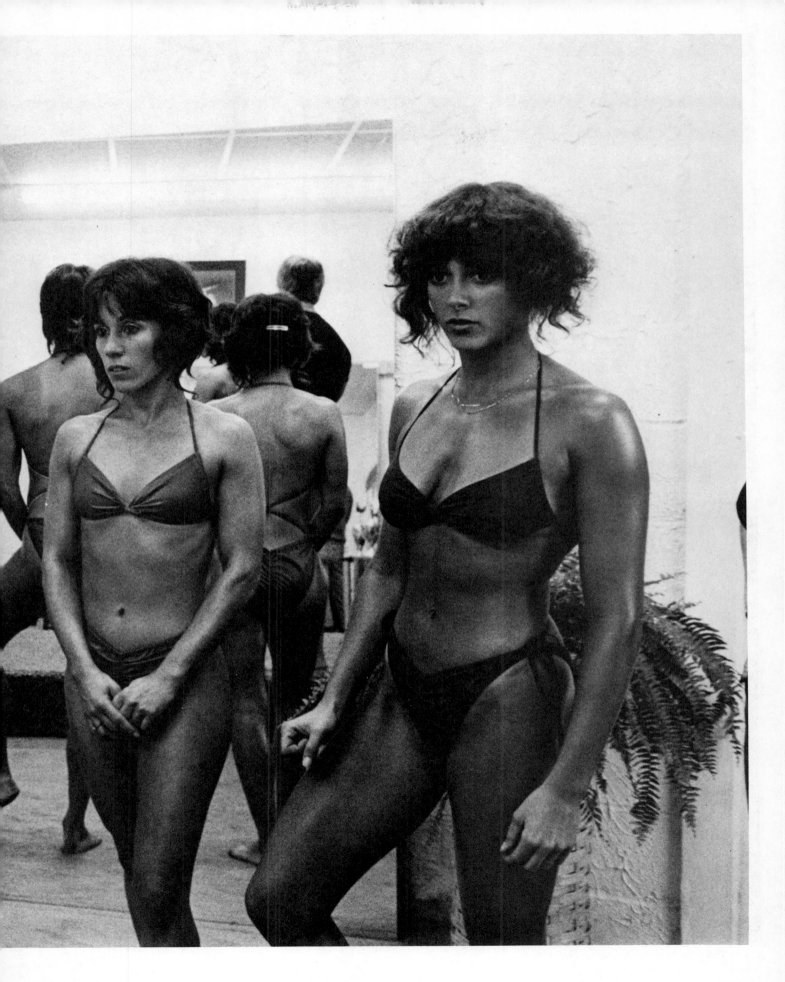

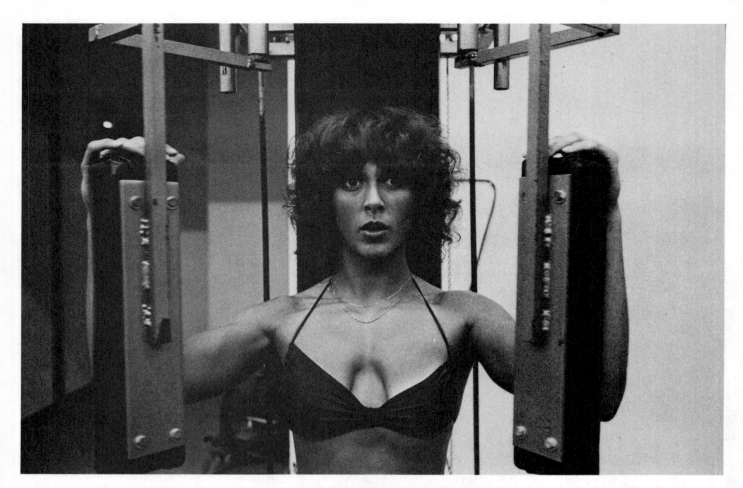

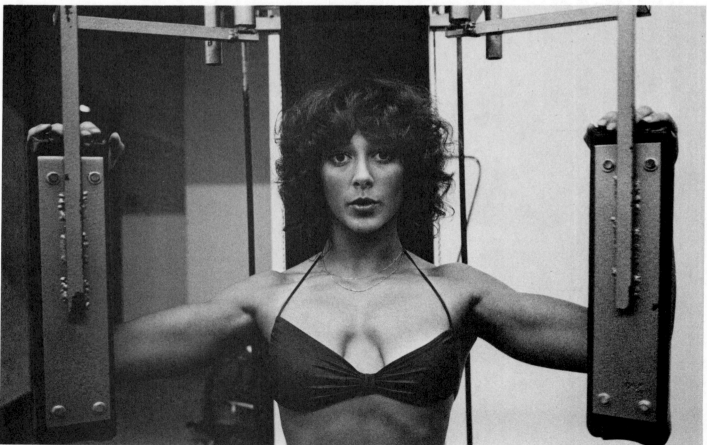

DeeDee Antonelli, working her chest

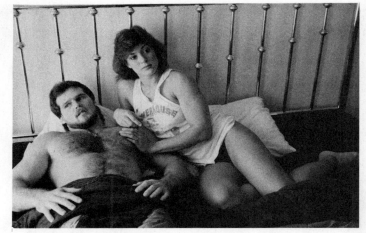

Lori Bowen and Randy Rice

of not looking womanly.

George Butler and I wanted to know more about DeeDee and Cindy, about their histories and ambitions, and what it felt like to be budding women bodybuilders. So when their workout was finished we asked them out for dinner. Before dinner we went back to our motel and talked. Cindy was dressed in black pants, a gray Playboy T-shirt, and a black satin jacket with "Pearson's Gym" on the back. Her look was both outrageous and witty in this working-class area on a January evening. DeeDee's look was neither, but with her wonderful body winking as she walked and her lovely, sultry face, she was as improbably loud-looking as Cindy was in the motel lobby, and together there they were as flashy as two enormous diamonds worn on the same hand.

DeeDee's real name was Deirdre. She was twenty years old, lived in Braintree, Massachusetts, was five feet five and a half inches tall, weighed one hundred ten pounds, and measured 36-23-35. She came from a close Italian family with four older brothers and an Italian chef for a father who has a penchant for garlic. She had graduated from high school, still lived at home, didn't have a steady boyfriend, and wanted to study nutrition and to become Miss Olympia. She had been training for a little over a year. She got interested in bodybuilding through a couple of her brothers who worked out, and quickly became more committed to it than either of them were. Her parents, she said, didn't like her bodybuilding—no one in her family had gone to the Miss Northeast, her only contest until then, and after it her mother wouldn't speak to her for three days. "They think it's a fad," she said, "something I'll get over." But she won't, she added.

DeeDee was not exactly sure how she had settled on bodybuilding to excel at, but it felt wonderfully natural to her. She loved the training, the posing, the good nutrition. She would never use drugs, she said, or train in a way that made her look less feminine, and

she believed she could get to the top of the sport without doing those things. But, much as she wanted to, getting to the top didn't *really* matter to her all that much. Along with her family and her schooling in nutrition, bodybuilding was her life, a big part of all she ever wanted to do with herself, and doing it, really, was its own reward.

With Cindy Hardee the question of getting to the top, like almost everything else, was a little more complicated than it was with DeeDee. She had not had a happy, conventional childhood or a loving, close-knit family. Like DeeDee she presently had no steady boyfriend and she had been training for a little over a year, but that was absolutely all the two women had in common. Cindy was twenty-four. Born in Jacksonville, Florida, she had had a miserable childhood and at fifteen she left home. She moved to New York, lived in a boardinghouse at first and then with an older man with whom she had "been affiliated" through her childhood, and took courses in dance and Japanese art. At sixteen she went back to Jacksonville and worked for a while as a landscaper and a carpenter's apprentice. Who knows if what all she says happened after that really happened? It is not uncommon for bodybuilders, male and female, to fiddle as creatively with their pasts as they do with their bodies. But I, for one, believe it did—partially because it seems to me an exactly perfect background for a female bodybuilder, and partially because no less exceptional a recent history could likely have left Cindy Hardee with the delighted ease she has with the world's randomness.

"As a carpenter's apprentice I was clearing three hundred dollars a week and my lady friends were making eighty-five dollars as secretaries. I bought myself a gold Seiko watch, I'll never forget it. I did dry-walls. I laid linoleum floors. I painted. I did masonry and I stayed in magnificent shape. It was very amusing.

"Then I met this gentleman, who was like thirty-three and I was seventeen. I had just graduated from beauty school, cosmetology school, got licensed and

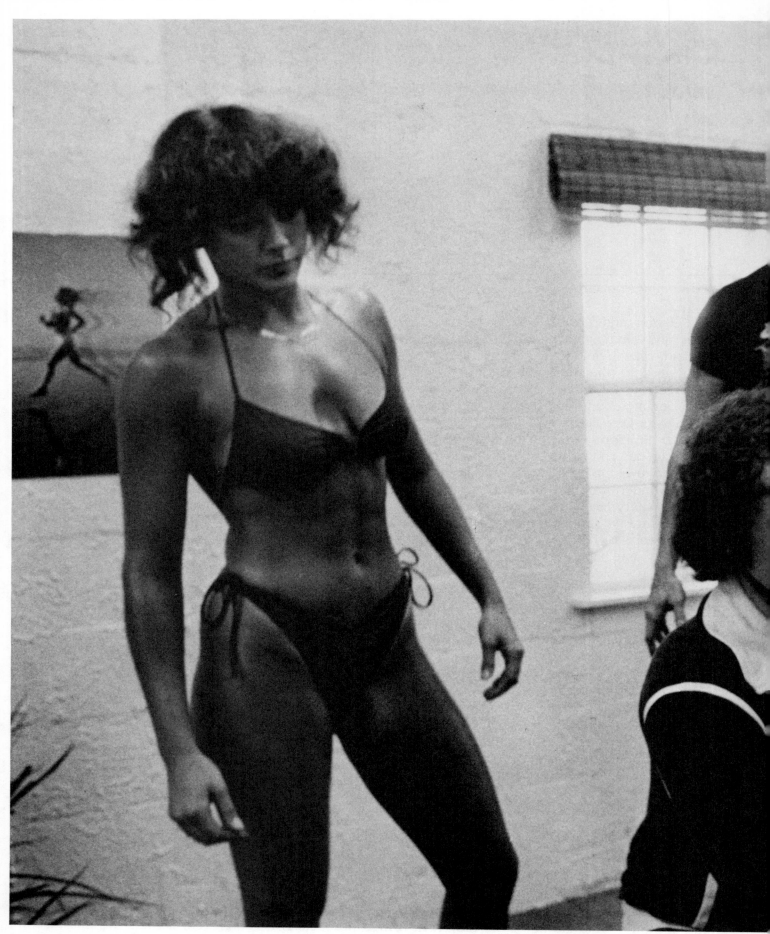

Stone at Work, Stone's Gym

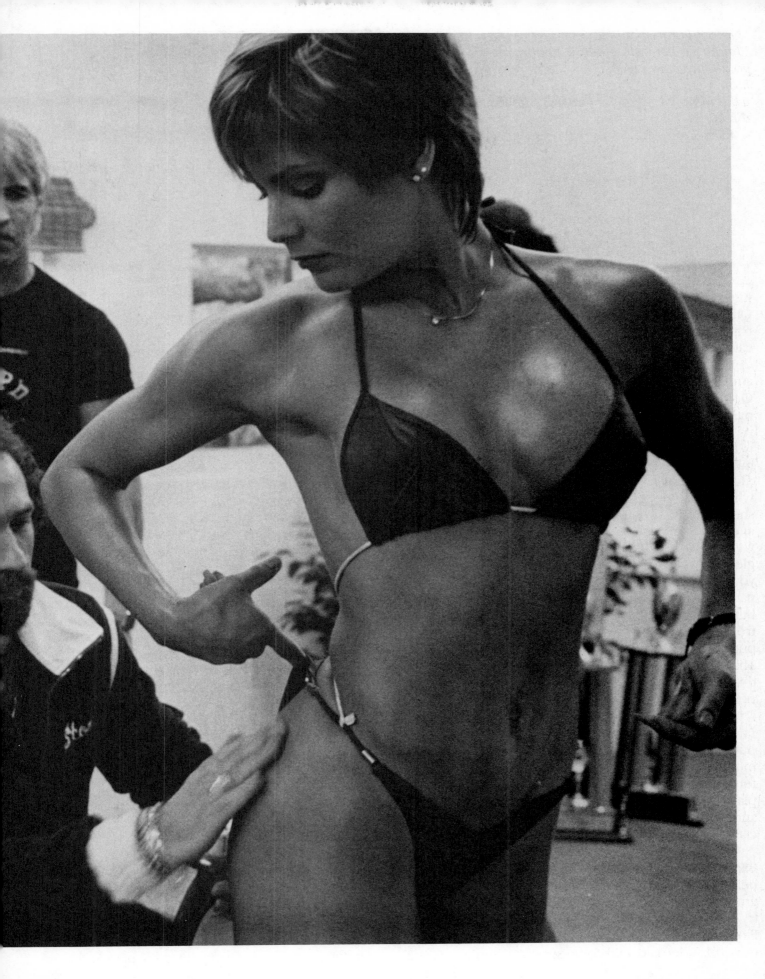

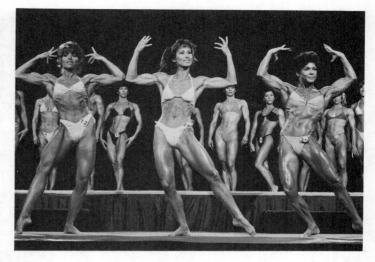

"I know I'm marketable. I know I've got a lot to offer. I know women relate to me. I know all this. How to go about getting it is different. I'm making good money now, but I know it's peanuts compared to what I know I could be making with the right direction."
—Rachel McLish

just wanted something to dabble in. My stepfather, Otto, is three time World Champion and two time European Champion in hair cutting. So this gentleman called me at work one day and said, 'What are you doing? Can you come to Orlando? I'm at Disney World and I'd love to see you.' He chartered me down to Orlando and I've been with him ever since until this past October. About seven years.

"We were living in New York, and one day I went with friends of mine who were auditioning for this big modeling agency. I had extremely long hair, down past my rear end and it was just beautiful. I pampered it my whole life long. And a lady came out of the office and she said to me, 'Yeah, you're the one we need for Long and Silky—come this way.' So I go to the office. 'What's your glove size?' I don't know, never owned a pair of gloves. They went right down the line. I was very young, I wrote my life away. They used me. I was a full page ad in *Cosmopolitan* at seventeen and made three hundred and fifty dollars a day for four days, shooting from ten to two. They did everything with me. They put me in everything—lingerie, costume jewelry. That's pretty much what caused us to travel as we did, this gentleman and I, because I needed to be in major ports to do my work.

"He had at that point some very good investments in oil with a buddy from Michigan, and he was in and out of the nightclub business. For a while we had more money than most people see in a lifetime and we afforded ourselves a lot of fun things. We had tons and played in the big league. Charter and Lear jets here and there, and diamonds and jewels. First class, all first class. It didn't last long, unfortunately.

"For a while we lived in a very small town called Barren Springs, Michigan, which was right in the fruit belt and on either side had a cherry orchard and grapes. It was magnificent—just being out in the country that I loved. From there we went back down to Florida and spent some time in Boca and further south in Fort Lauderdale. Did some serious gambling. Came

back up to Jacksonville, got a very good job with a local sports merchandiser that had me doing all the merchandise marts—Miami, New York, Chicago, Atlanta— wearing their goods. I was their live model. I enjoyed that a lot. I like being with people.

"In early seventy-five we lived in Gloucester in a beautiful home. We were fortunate enough to have rented an island which is one hundred acres, thirty different species of birds, red fox, silver fox, deer, all kinds of wildlife. It was a sanctuary. It was a very memorable time in my life. I'll never forget it. I still dream about the sunrises and sunsets I saw there . . ."

It goes on—more of Florida, back to the south shore of Massachusetts; some high living, some low; finally meeting Lenny Archambault through his friend the gentleman and starting to train seriously and finally breaking up with the gentleman. And now here she was, at twenty-four, five feet six, one hundred ten pounds at contest weight, 39-20-30, smoking and drinking and wisecracking up a storm, still as much on the make for life, as eager for its possibilities and as unwearied by them as she was at fifteen, and still creating herself by nobody's pattern but her own. Cindy *believed* that she would soon win the Olympia and be picked up for endorsements by a major manufacturer, that she would act for a while and make lots of money again, and then marry happily and have six little girls, one a year for six years. She believed all that would happen, but if it didn't, if life didn't get her to all those places, she was sure as hell going to enjoy the ride anyway. I asked Cindy what her five favorite things were.

Waking up, sex, food, fast cars and money, she said, and with that remembered that she was hungry.

The four of us went to an Italian restaurant in Braintree. We learned at the door that the place took neither credit cards nor checks, and none of us had enough cash to eat on. "No problem," said Cindy, leading the way in. "We'll figure something out."

We sat in a booth made for two people in the

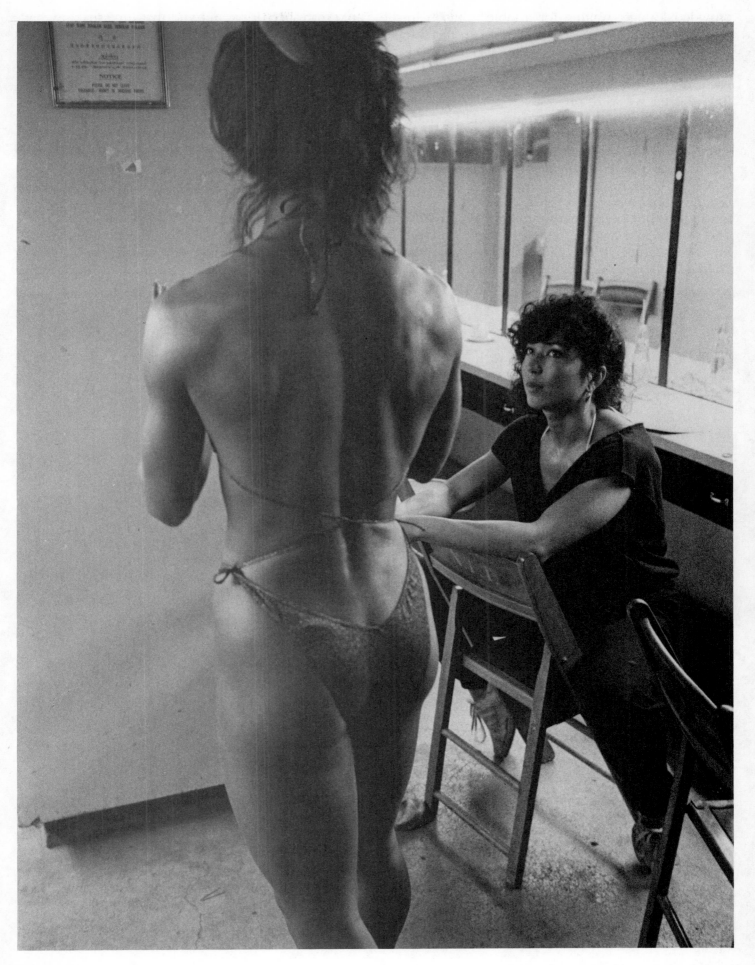

crowded lounge, waiting for a table to open in the dining room. Seated at the bar across from us was a tired-looking middle-aged couple, also waiting for a table. They looked short-tempered and unhappy with each other, and at first they seemed grateful for the loud theater we were providing. Sitting on my lap in the narrow booth, her legs crossed and the pant leg pulled up over one of her wonderful calves, Cindy smoked and drank with appetite and mentioned loudly that she entertained lascivious fantasies about Walter Cronkite. The couple at the bar stared at her, at all of us, and smiled nervously. Cindy and DeeDee went on to say that they both fantasized about Johnny Carson. The woman and man at the bar looked at each other for the first time in ten minutes. Cindy sucked on a

lime from her drink and said that lime-sucking made the stomach contract and was a good thing to do just before competition. She asked me if I wanted to know a funny thing: As an embryo, she said, she had had the heartbeat of a man. *That* should have told her something.

"What do you people do?" asked the man at the bar, his eyes flitting back and forth strangely between the two eye-popping women in the booth. I explained that Misses Hardee and Antonelli were female body-builders, and that Butler and I were journalists doomed to their company in order to observe and report them.

The man looked gloomily at Cindy sitting on my lap. "Just making the best of it, huh?" he said.

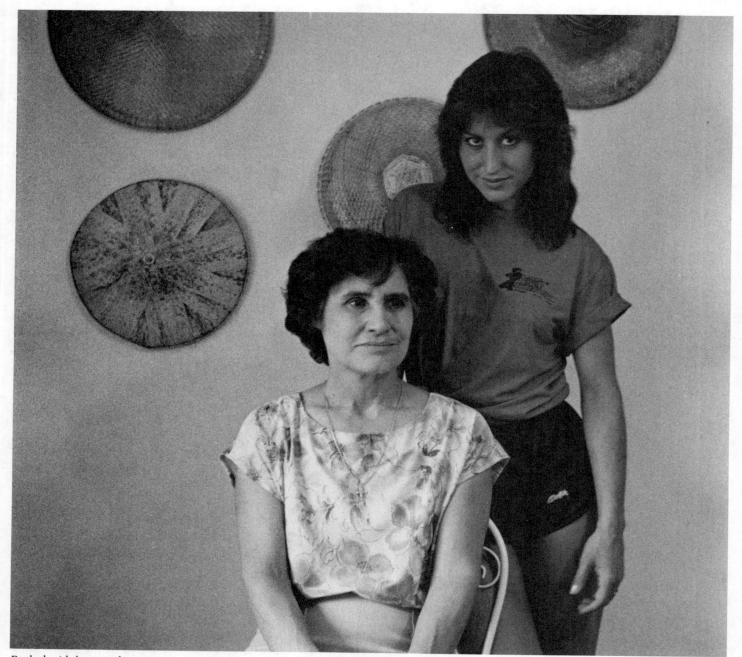

Rachel with her mother

The eyes of the woman at the bar had taken on a hostile glaze. "Women bodybuilders . . . *God*. Like, what do you eat?"

"Skinless, boneless chicken breasts cooked only in white wine, no salt," said Cindy Hardee gaily, hooking my foot with hers and polishing off her drink. "And nothing else."

A waiter came in and told us our table was ready. The two women bodybuilders stood up and walked off, with George and me following, toward a big meal without knowing or caring how the bill would be paid, and every eye in the lounge was on them. At the door I turned around to look at the man and woman at the bar. I suppose I was expecting "Who was that masked man?" expressions on their faces—slightly awed, puz- zled expressions, reflecting some vision of the future they might have just had, the cheering vision of some strange new freedom. But they were only bitching at each other.

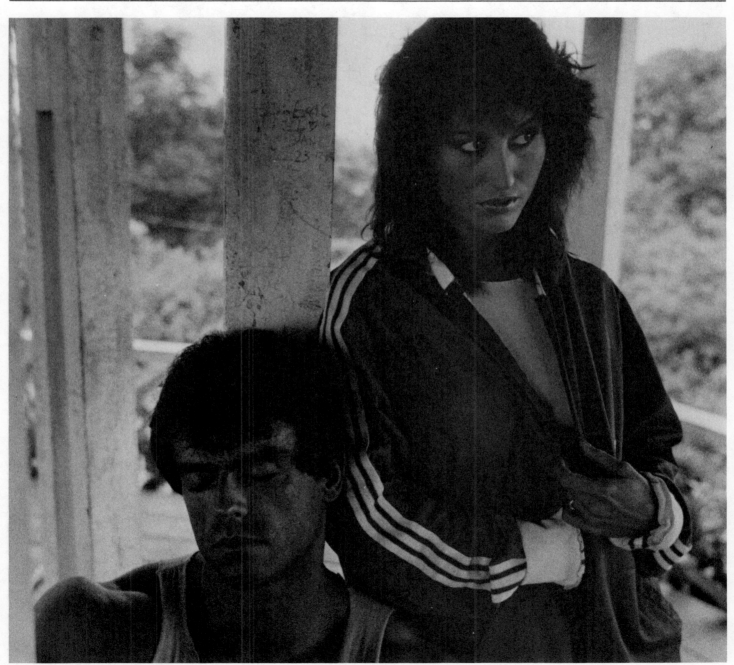

Rachel with Christian Janatsch

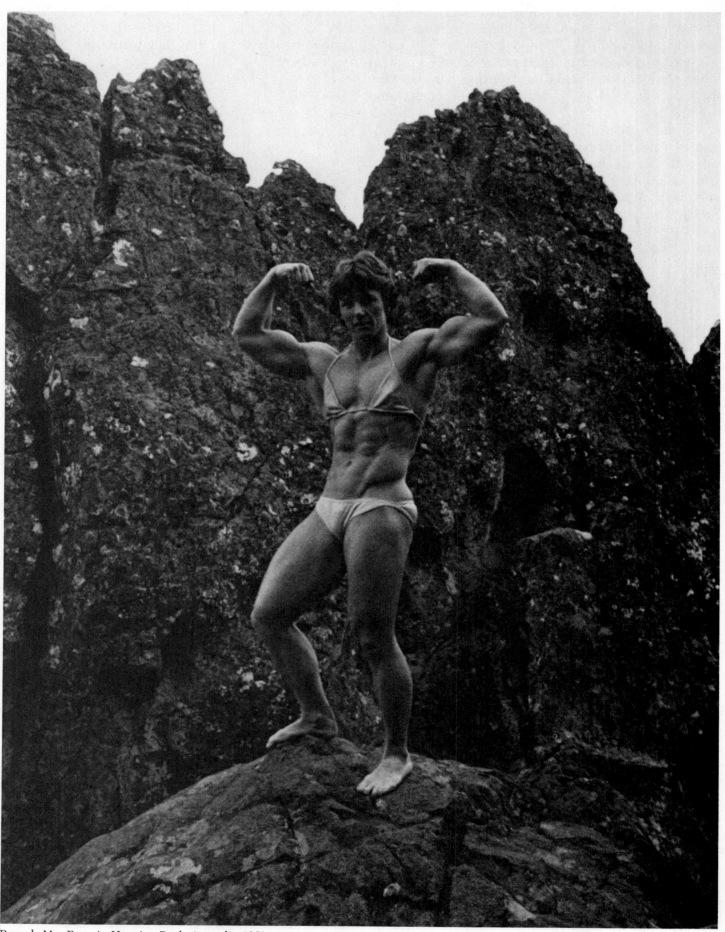

Beverly May Francis, Hanging Rock, Australia, 1983

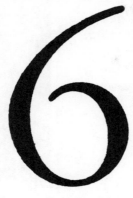

George Butler and I wanted to make one more trip. We felt that our effort to describe competitive female bodybuilding by characterizing the spectrum of women who participate in it was missing something. If Cindy Hardee was at one end of that spectrum, who or what was at the other end?

In early 1983 Wayne DeMilia found a picture that provided a clue. It was a small photograph, published in a Canadian bodybuilding book. The caption claimed the subject was a woman, but though her posing suit clearly included a bikini bra, your eyes told you this person *had* to be a man. No woman could have thighs like that, your eyes said, or shoulders or arms like that, not to mention the abdominal muscles. No woman has a stomach like that, your eyes insisted: it has to be a man dressed, for some weird reason, like a woman.

But it wasn't. It was an authentic woman. Her name was Bev Francis, and George and I thought we saw in her the other end of our spectrum. To be certain, we would have to travel to Melbourne, Australia, where she lived, and in June 1983 that is what we did.

Though she is almost certainly the most muscular woman alive—and very possibly the most muscular woman who ever lived—Bev Francis is not officially a bodybuilder. As of the summer of 1983 she had never competed in a bodybuilding contest and she did not develop her muscles for the sake of having them or showing them off. Rather, her truly astounding muscularity is the by-product of the training she has done for what is an equally astounding athletic career. She is now twenty-eight. She started training seriously for sports when she was nineteen, at the University of Melbourne, and since that time she has put the shot, thrown the discus and the javelin, sprinted and power-lifted—all at, or very near, world-class levels. For the past five years she has been the number-two female Australian shot-putter, as well as one of the country's leading female javelin and discus throwers. But her best sport is power-lifting, and in that she has no fe-

male peer anywhere in the world.

World championships in power-lifting for women have been held for only the past four years, and Bev has won her weight-class in each of those championships, competing twice in the 165-pound class and twice in the 181-pound class. Power-lifting competition consists of three lifts—the squat, the bench-press, and the dead-lift—each a pure and demanding measure of a particular type of physical strength. Within a given weight-class, the winner of a power-lifting contest is whoever lifts the highest total amount of weight in all three lifts. Bev holds six individual power-lifting world records—the squat, the bench-press and the total in the 165-pound class, and the squat, bench and total in the 181-pound class—and her total in the 181-pound class in last year's championship, 577½ kilograms (1,270 pounds), is the highest ever achieved by a woman in *any* weight-class, including the super-heavy. In fact, that total is so high that it could win the 181-pound class of some male power-lifting competitions.

In the bench-press, you lie flat on your back on a bench and use the muscles of your chest, shoulders and triceps to push a bar loaded with weight off your chest and upward until your arms are locked. Bev's personal best at this lift is 331 pounds. In the squat, you stand with the bar held on your shoulders behind your neck, squat down until your upper legs are parallel with the floor, then use your thigh and lower back muscles to stand up straight again. Bev has squatted with 480 pounds. A dead-lift is simply that—the dead-lifting of a bar off the floor and standing up with it until the back is straight. The lift is made with muscles in the legs, lower back, shoulders and arms. Bev's best dead-lift is 476 pounds.

Taken together these lifts test practically every major muscle group in the body, and the strength necessary to do them all well is a complete, brute strength at pulling and pushing and standing up under a load—a strength with few subtleties and one that is rarely if ever associated with women. There are many, many

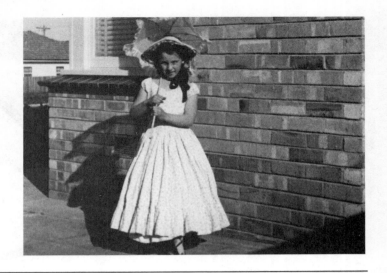

big men—bodybuilders, wrestlers, professional football players—men known for their strength, with eighteen-inch arms and way upwards of two hundred pounds of heft, who have sweated and grunted with iron for years without ever bench-pressing 331 pounds, squatting 480, or dead-lifting 476. Yet those lifts have all been made (in each case at a bodyweight of 178 pounds or less) by a five-foot-five-inch *woman*.

A woman with more brute strength than all but a very few men? What could such a creature be like? I showed Bev's picture to an English computer programmer sitting next to me on the long flight to Australia. He stared at the picture sadly for a long time and shook his head.

"You Americans started all this," he said, "with your bloody feminism and all. God knows where *this* is going to lead us."

I wanted to tell him something I had not said to anyone yet. I wanted to try out the fact objectively—get it out there and try to get some sane, cheerful handle on it before I arrived in Melbourne.

"I am six foot two and two hundred pounds," I said. "I have been lifting weights for twenty years. This woman is stronger than I am."

"Right," said the Englishman, going back to his book. "Well, you can't say you people didn't ask for it."

At the outermost limit of any human continuum one can generally look forward to finding some sort of monster. In that respect, Bev Francis is a disappointment. Her appearance, to be sure, is not traditionally female, but neither is it monstrously male. Her weight when I met her was down to 158 from the 180 pounds at which she had competed in the last women's powerlifting championship. At that lighter weight, dressed in jeans and a short-sleeved shirt, with her short hair and broad shoulders, her bulging arms and thighs and her narrow hips, she looks from a distance like a stocky, well-developed boy—a farm boy, maybe, who muscles a tractor around, eats well, and lifts a lot of hay. But up close, she is obviously and appealingly a woman. Though her hair is short, it is soft, wavy, and well tended. She has dainty hands with tapered fingers and nails, a pretty mouth, and gray-blue, one-hundred-percent female eyes that are smart, sympathetic and easily amused. Her face overall is a strong one, with a prominent nose and a long jaw. It is a forthright face that expresses much of her personality, an unlikely mixture of vulnerability and stone-solid self-confidence, curiosity and discipline, self-containment and ambition. When you meet Bev Francis, shake her hand and talk to her for a while, you know without a doubt that you are dealing with a female, but a female with a sharp male edge that cuts its own track. Her muscles aside, there is very little about her that could be read as cuddly or dependent. Inside and out, she is well-knit, compact and forceful.

After lunch on the day I met her we went over to the place that occupies the center of her life. That place is a small section of the University of Melbourne campus, and within it Bev has both dream and reality. Her friends are there, her work and her play are there, many of her ambitions are there, and a particular man is there who is at once her coach, her friend, her adviser, her surrogate father, and her father confessor. The man's name is Franz Stampfl, and he sits in a wheelchair inside an athletic hut at the center of the center of Bev Francis's life. Within a few hundred yards of the hut is the gym where she works out, the track she runs on, the fields where she puts the shot and throws the javelin and discus—and those places are usually crowded with her closest friends. Until recently there was practically nothing Bev Francis wanted that could not be found within a few hundred yards of Franz's hut. But during the past few months she has decided to become the world's best female bodybuilder. Even for Bev Francis that will take a lot of doing, and much of that doing will have to be done a long way from here.

The hut is a small two-room building, built as an

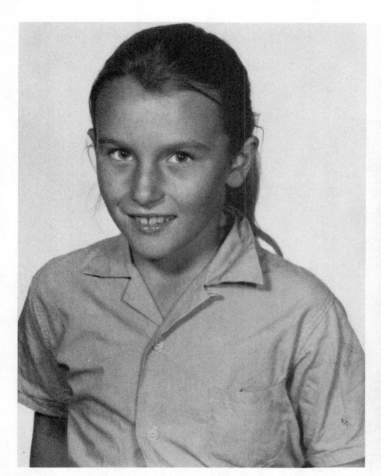

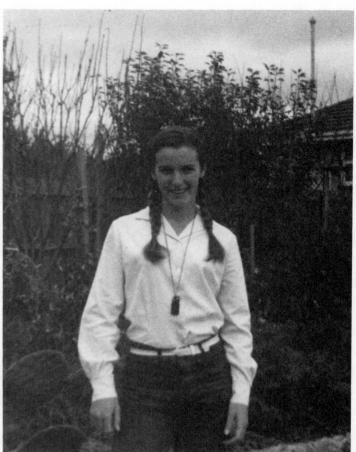

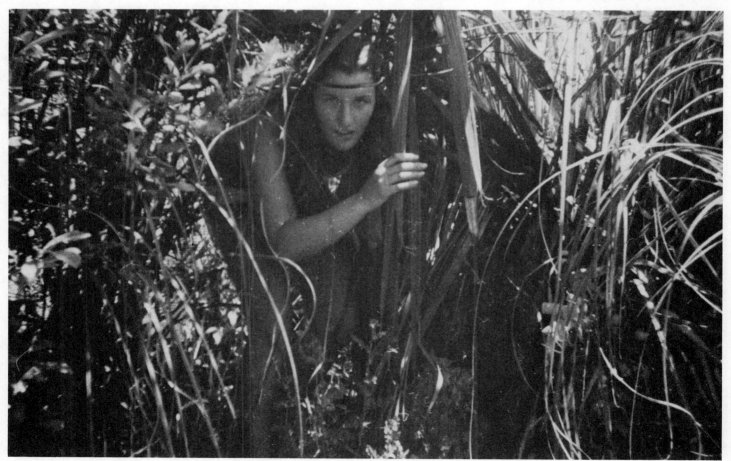

Bev Francis as a girl

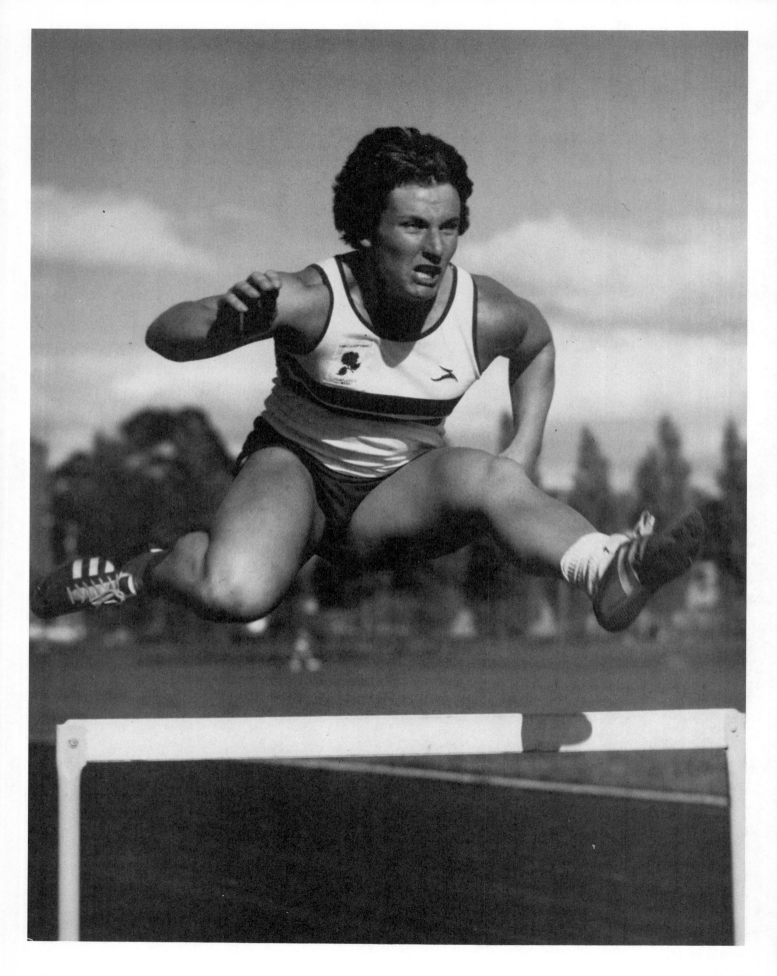

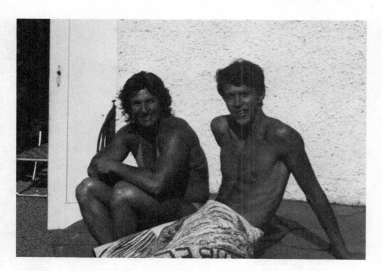

office for Franz by the University of Melbourne. From it he supervises one of the most unusual and effective track and field programs in the world. Inside there is a large closet full of shotputs, javelins and footballs; a whole wall of shelves full of sneakers and training clothes; a finch in a cage; a radio which is always broadcasting Australian football matches; a small icebox full of juices and tonic water; and a few pieces of old, comfortable furniture. Hung on the walls are posters of big, strong women putting the shot, running, ski racing and power-lifting; there is also a lettered sign that reads: "I SUPPORT WOMEN'S SPORTS," and another that says, "THE UPPER CRUST IS A LOT OF CRUMBS STICKING TOGETHER."

Franz Stampfl sits in his wheelchair in the middle of the smaller of the two rooms talking to Bev, who sits across from him on a couch. Athletes, most of them women, come and go, and there are usually four or five sitting around at any given time during the two to three hours Franz is there every day. They talk to him and listen—mostly listen, for Franz has a lot to say. Most of what he has had to say to Bev recently concerns her becoming a bodybuilder. Having the athlete's usual low regard for bodybuilding, he is not enthusiastic. But since she is determined to do it anyway, he wants her to go into her first contest (in Las Vegas, December 1983) more muscular than anyone has ever before seen a woman. He wants her to blow the "skinned rabbits"—as he calls the lithe, pretty women who presently dominate the sport in America —right off the stage with *big,* uncompromised muscles.

"You be who you are," he tells Bev. "You cannot play their game. To *hell* with sex appeal—this is too important. You go there and show them who you are. You make your statement. You show them something they have never seen before."

Franz *means* this. He talks to Bev in a profoundly intimate, proprietary way, and you know even before you are told that the statement he wants made in Las

Vegas is his as much as it is hers. In fact, it has been his for a very long time.

Franz is sixty-nine. He has been an ardent supporter of women's rights since the 1920s, when as a teenager in Austria he worked to decriminalize abortion in that country. When he moved to England in 1937 and began coaching track and field there, he saw no reason not to coach women along with men—despite a worldwide disregard at that time for women in sports —and he has been doing that ever since. In 1939, well known and respected in England as a coach, he was nevertheless interned by the British along with other German and Austrian nationalists and was shipped in chains to Australia to wait out the war in prison. But the Australians let him out of jail to join the army. In 1946 he was discharged from the Australian army, and he married and moved back to England. During the next nine years in both England and Northern Ireland, Stampfl established himself as one of the top track and field coaches in the British Isles. He coached at Cambridge, began a national coaching system for Northern Ireland, and in 1954 he coached Roger Bannister to the world's first four-minute mile. In 1955, Franz moved back to Australia to take a senior lectureship and coaching position at the University of Melbourne. Since then he has turned one hundred eighty women and men into Australian national champions at various track and field events, and he has coached at least one national champion in every track and field event there is. It is likely that no other track and field coach in the world can match that record of success on a national level. In addition, he has seen Bev and quite a few others of his athletes go on to successful world competition.

Franz was himself an accomplished athlete—a champion ski racer, a sprinter, jumper, hurdler and javelin thrower—who at sixty-five could still bench-press 250 pounds. Then two and a half years ago, his car was run into from behind while he was stopped at a traffic light, and he was left a quadriplegic. The acci-

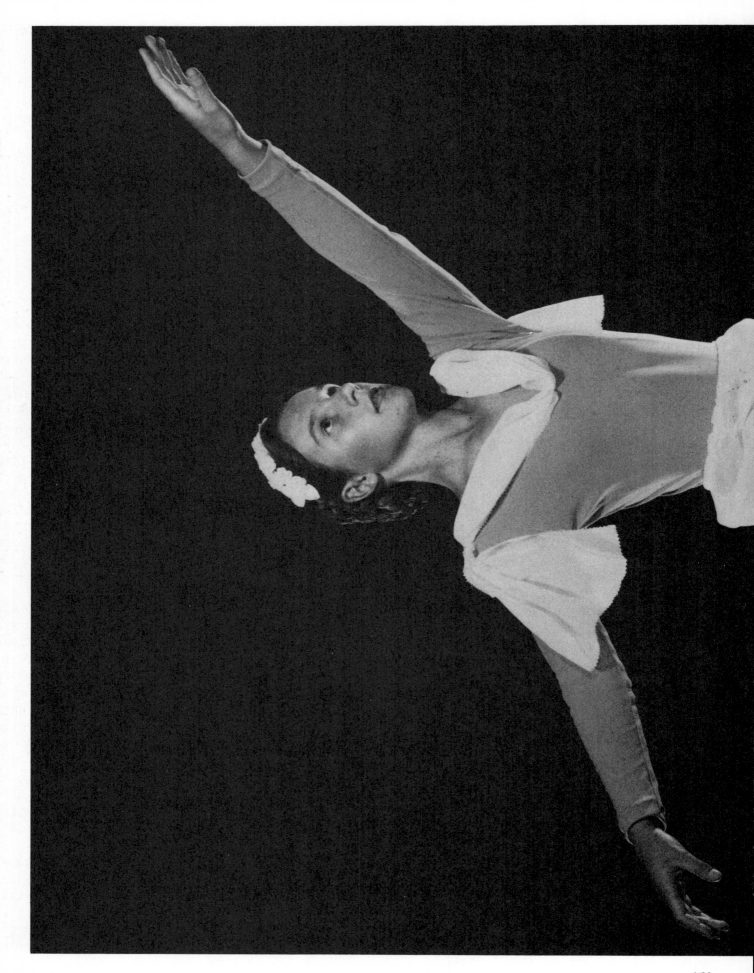

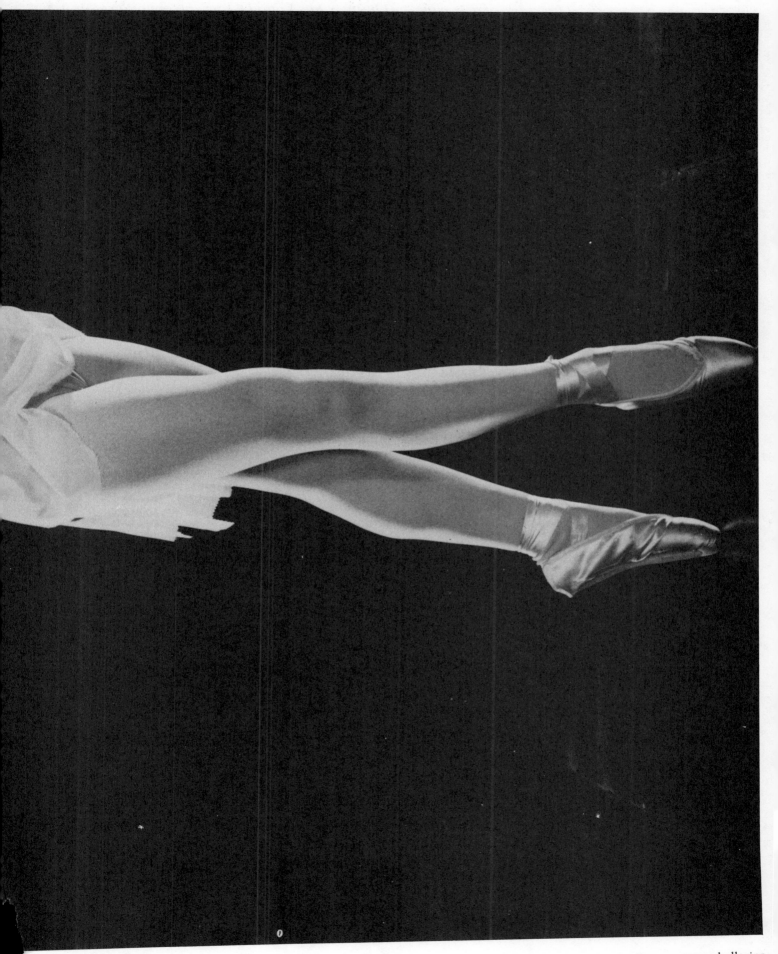

Bev as a young ballerina

151

"I feel very much a woman. I feel more of a woman now than before I started training by far. I feel that I've developed my personality as a woman to a much greater degree. I may have thrown away some of the traditional aspects of femininity as we are brought up in society to believe or accept, but that's not a bad thing. I don't like being told exactly what I've got to be like. If I'm not like that, why should I constantly try and fit in to somebody else's arbitrary feminine role? I don't miss being thought of as silly, giggly, useless, incapable. All of those things I don't miss at all. I find a woman who fits into all of those stereotypes of femininity very boring, and a person that I don't want to associate with. I can wear a dress as often as I like, but I don't find them very comfortable. My way of life is an active one and in a dress you can't sit down and put your feet up, you can't do cartwheels, you can't go and jump over a fence. You can't walk in lots of places in high heels. I believe in comfort and in things that allow you to do the things you want to do. . . . I have female sex organs, I have female responses, I have female hormones in my body, female chromosomes, or whatever. I can't change that and I don't want to. I'm happy with being a woman, and I'm very happy with my female responses."
—Bev Francis

---

dent did not stop his coaching, though his position at the university is no longer an official one. Between fifty and sixty male and female athletes still train under his supervision. He sets their schedules in his hut and drives his wheelchair out to watch them run, throw and lift. Over twenty percent of those athletes are women, and it is with those women athletes that he is most involved. His training methods for them, he says, are exactly the same as they are for men. After training over twenty thousand athletes in his career, he believes that women are inherently equal to men athletically; the fact that that equality is rarely recognized or acknowledged outside of Melbourne is due, he believes, to various environmental factors that continue to work against all women involved in competitive sports. Not the least of those factors, according to Franz, is old-fashioned male chauvinism, particularly among coaches.

"Most coaches in America think it is sissy to train women," he says. "Everywhere in the world men create pressure against women developing themselves into all they can be."

There is certainly no such pressure here in Franz's hut. Women becoming all they can be are everywhere. One such woman, named Sue, comes into the hut while Franz is talking to Bev. Sue is nearly six feet tall and looks as if she weighs close to two hundred pounds, most of which is carried in her astonishingly muscular legs. Dressed in leotards, she has been running 50-meter wind-sprints on the cinder track outside as part of her training program for shot-putting. Though she has only recently taken up the sport, she is already one of the top-ranked women shot-putters in the country. She sits shyly in a corner of the room, her great Percheron haunches resting lightly on the edge of a chair, listening to every word Franz says. After a while—acting, it appears, on intuition—she walks across the room and holds a glass up to Franz's face. As he does at frequent intervals during the day, the coach interrupts his conversation long enough to sip some gin and tonic through a straw.

Within a few minutes another female athlete comes into the hut, this one a pretty Australian Olympic giant slalom skier named Jenny. She too sits and listens, and periodically holds up the glass of gin and tonic for Franz to drink.

During the time I am there a half-dozen of these women come into the hut, sit for a while, and leave again to resume training for the javelin, the discus and the shotput, for running, jumping, skiing, and powerlifting. All of them are inordinately muscular and intent, and most of them are enormous. It is oddly dislocating. Franz says of his long dedication to female self-actualization that he is "a coach with a social conscience," but that doesn't begin to cover it. After an hour or two inside his hut you can easily come to feel that you are in the middle of an enchantment, a fairy tale about happy Amazons, and that Franz Stampfl is in fact a coach with a magic wand.

Bev Francis and her best friend, Gail Mulhall, are lifting weights together in the Richmond Football Club Gym. Gail, who under Franz's coaching has become the best female shot-putter in Australia and one of the best in the world, is also a power-lifter who won the 198-pound weight division at this year's world championships. She is the Puck of Franz's Amazons—a huge, bright-humored, effervescent woman who keeps the others energized and laughing. She has just recently been married, and her husband, Nigel, an ex-Olympic lifter, is one of the four or five men working out in the gym alongside Gail, Bev and three or four other women.

Men and women using a gym at the same time is not uncommon in the U.S. anymore, but men and women actually *training* together is almost unheard of. There are usually a number of good reasons for that, the main one being that in the States men almost universally train differently than women, using heavier weights and doing more serious strength exercise

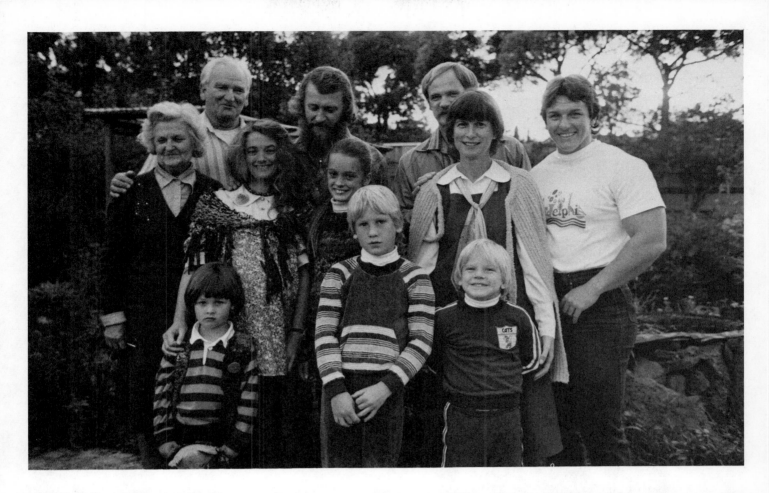

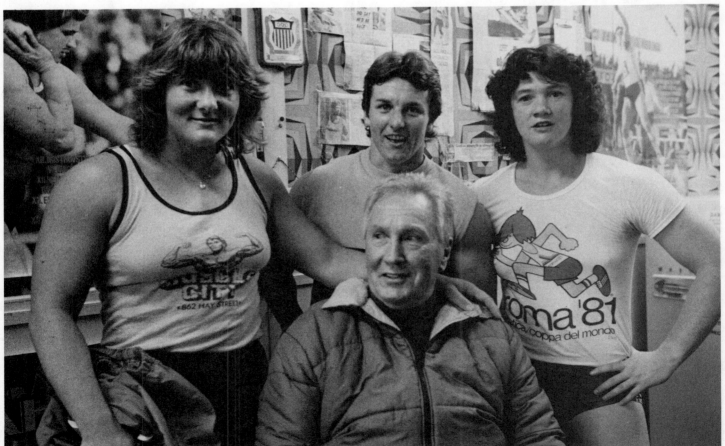

With Franz Stampfl and fellow athletes

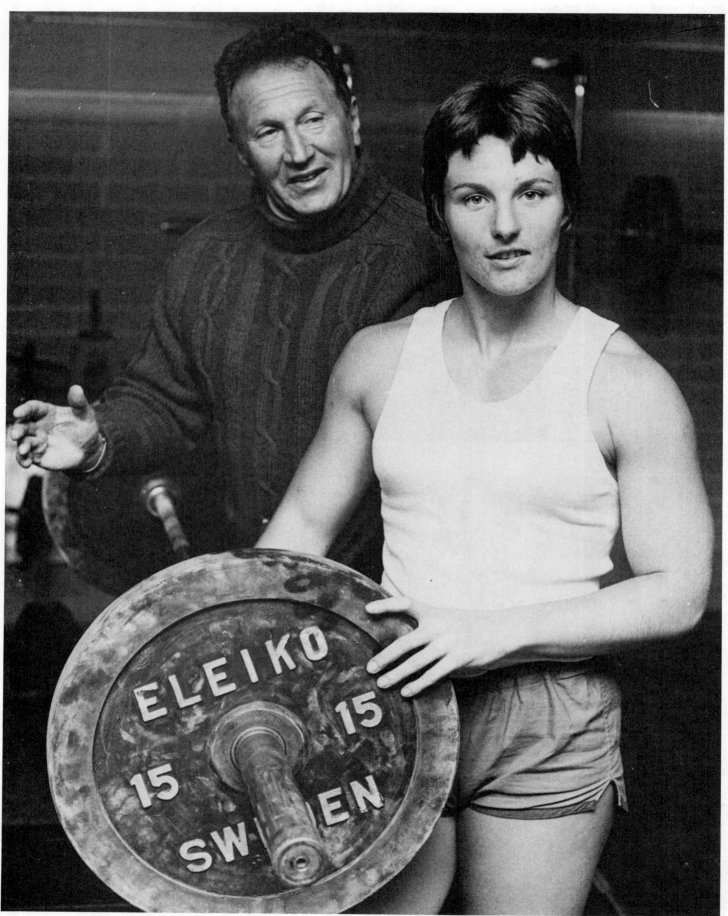

Bev and Franz, the early days

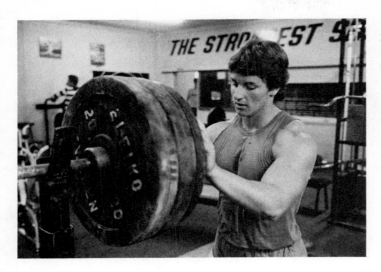

The majority of American women bodybuilders (a group which could be expected to use weights as seriously as anyone) train almost delicately, doing shaping exercises with light weights, often without breaking a sweat and practically never to the point of real pain or muscular exhaustion. But here in the Richmond Football Club Gym pain and exhaustion are the natural and desired ends of weight training for women as well as for men, and since the women here are as strong as all but the strongest men, co-ed training is customary and unselfconscious.

The gym itself is a long ground-level room stuffed with old free-weights, a Nautilus leg machine, a decrepit multistation weight machine, punching bags, medicine balls and a mini-tramp. It is a serious, old-fashioned gym with few mirrors, no chrome, and the layered, acidic smell of decades of expended muscular effort—the good smell of an old lifting belt. Bev is doing super-sets for her upper legs, going from a set of leg-presses on the Nautilus machine to leg-extensions to squats without resting between the sets, and doing each set "to exhaustion," or until she can't manage another repetition. It is a brutally painful workout, as tough as they come for a woman or a man, and light-years tougher than any leg training I've seen American female bodybuilders do.

Bev moans through the end of a super-set, gulping for air and standing up with one last rep as Gail and the others shout encouragement. She clangs the bar into the squat rack and walks around the gym grimacing and shaking out her thighs. Those thighs are each twenty-four inches around, only five inches less than her waist, and flare dramatically along their outside edges. Her legs are storybook legs, the legs of a centaur or of Diana, with cleanly divided slabs of interlocking muscle tapering to the knees, sweeping outward at the calves and narrowing again quickly to the ankles; and, like other parts of her body, they bear so little resemblance to normal twentieth-century female structure that a common response to the shock of encountering them, either in photographs or in the flesh, is to insist that they must be, in effect, fake—the synthetic product of drug use.

But the fact is that while anabolic, or growth-enhancing, drugs such as steroids are used by some female track and field athletes, power-lifters and bodybuilders the use of those drugs by no means guarantees achievement. If steroids alone could produce an Arnold Schwarzenegger or a Bev Francis, there would be thousands of them walking the streets of every city in the world. Bev's musculature is unique among contemporary women, and no uniqueness comes cheaply. In her case it is the result of good genes and years of unrelenting work. In the small two-room flat where she lives, she keeps a diary which has recorded in it every day of her training since November 6, 1976. The diary consists of five filled notebooks, with the sixth one almost completed. It records in exact detail the shot-putting workouts, sprinting, distance running, jumping exercises, discus and javelin workouts, starts out of blocks, bodybuilding training, power- and Olympic-lifting, bicycling and swimming (when she is too injured or sick to do anything else) that she has done over the past seven years, and there is no chemical smell whatsoever to those pages. They smell like nothing more than sweat.

Here is a sample entry, for May 13, 1979:

One-half mile walk to Como. Pulse 50. Four-mile run at Como. Pulse 122 to 62 in one minute. Did Como exercises. One and one-half mile warmup. Five sprint starts from blocks with 30 meter runs. 200 meter time-trial in 26.4 seconds. Weights: bench-press—10 x 100, 10 x 120, 10 x 140, 10 x 160. Squats—10 x 132, 10 x 154, 10 x 168, 10 sets of 5 reps at 198 pounds. Arm curls—four sets of 10 with 25-pound dumbbells. Reverse wrist curls—four sets of 10 with 25-pound barbell. Wrist curls—four sets of 10 with 35-pound barbell. Straight arm pulleys—four sets of 10 with 60. Situps—one set of 100. Front dumbbell presses (inclined)—one set of 10 with 45-pound dumbbells. Body

"People often mistake me for a man, which I can understand because of the shoulders and very short haircut. People were just brought up to superficially look at people, and assume by their appearances what they are. The obvious things happen. I go into women's toilets and people say, 'Excuse me, do you realize that this is a ladies' room?' and I say, 'Of course I do.' People have asked me whether I was a male or a female and I've said female and they've refused to believe it. They say, no you're not. That really irritates me because I'm an honest person. But I try not to show my anger with them because aggression is a male characteristic and that's exactly what they expect, so I try very hard to control my temper, so that I don't once again feed into another slot they see as a stereotype. They've already seen the strong-looking body, so I don't want to show them something else that they think is male to back up their belief. I have to be very, very controlled, very careful what I say to people."
—Bev Francis

weight: 71.6 kilos (157 pounds). Total weight lifted for workout: 28,820 pounds. Total distance run: 5¾ miles.

I counted the days Bev had missed working out, for travel or ill health, over a period of five years. There were fewer than seventy. There is no drug known that can supply you with that much taste for work, and it is work that has made her body what it is.

Here at the gym today she is doing power-lifting, rather than bodybuilding, work for the Victorian Power-lifting Championships that are coming up soon, and that means she is training more for strength than for shape and definition. But she has begun to add bodybuilding exercises to her routine, and by the middle of the summer she will switch over to a pure bodybuilding schedule and begin to "cut up" for meeting Rachel and Kike and the others at the Caesar's Palace World Cup competition in Las Vegas in December.

Despite what Franz has advised, she knows that size alone won't win that contest for her and she wants badly to win it, both for her sake and for Franz's. To do that, to become the first truly muscular woman to win a major U.S. bodybuilding championship, she will have to be almost flawlessly defined and symmetrical as well as muscular, and she will have to pose well. All of that is a tall order for someone who has never before trained for bodybuilding or entered a bodybuilding competition, but Bev believes she can accomplish it, and she believes she will win the contest. Hard work is nothing new to her, and neither is perseverance. And, though she has not always had it, neither is self-confidence.

When she first met Franz Stampfl, Bev Francis was nineteen and he was sixty, and there was nothing about her to suggest to either of them that she would become one of the most extraordinary female athletes in the world. She was a conventional-looking teenager from a conventional background. Neither of her parents nor any of her four older siblings was particularly athletic. She had played sports in school, but not ex-

ceptionally well, and she had been a ballet dancer since age four, but not an exceptionally good one. But Bev had always thought of herself as being special, she had always admired strength, and she wanted badly, when she entered the University of Melbourne and met Franz, to *do* something with her life. When Franz told her she could become a first-rate athlete she didn't believe him. Over the next few years he helped her to believe in herself and, in the process, to begin to become all that she might be.

"As I started my athletics, Franz was the person who said to me, 'You can be a Victorian champion, a state champion.' And I said, 'That's rubbish.' He said, 'I know you've got it, and I know you can do it.' I had no belief in myself. He had tons of it. He had enough to give me my share too. He kept pushing, he kept encouraging, and just holding me up with his whole idea that women should do this sort of work, that they look better when they are muscular, and that I was looking better the more muscular I got. But he wouldn't let me lose my femininity. I didn't lose anything as a woman and that was very important. You don't want to lose your sexuality. Especially at nineteen, going into your twenties, and he built up my sexuality, my own belief in my sexuality, and my belief in myself as a whole person, as a woman. That included the weight-lifting; it included getting stronger and more muscular. If he hadn't encouraged me in that way and given me the belief in myself, I would never have had the courage to throw away those traditional aspects of femininity and develop this new way of life."

The staggering work of that new way of life, along with Franz's urgings and Bev's growing confidence in the self she was becoming, made her into not only a world-class athlete but a physical oddity—a woman who more than once has been turned out of a ladies' room and has otherwise routinely been mistaken for a man. In becoming the strongest female power-lifter in the world she has also become the world's most mus-

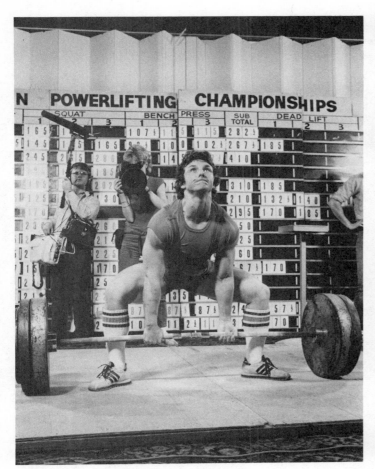
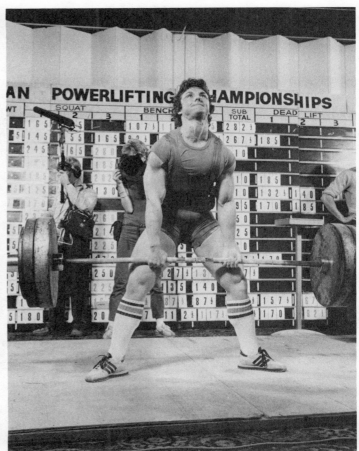
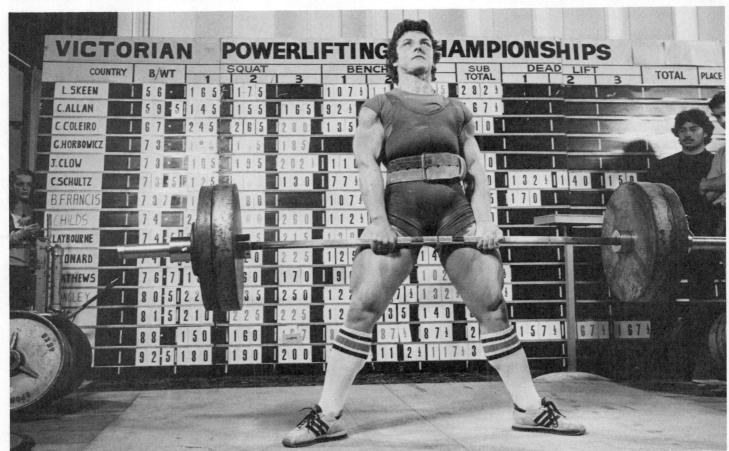

Bev winning Victorian Powerlifting Championships, Melbourne, 1983

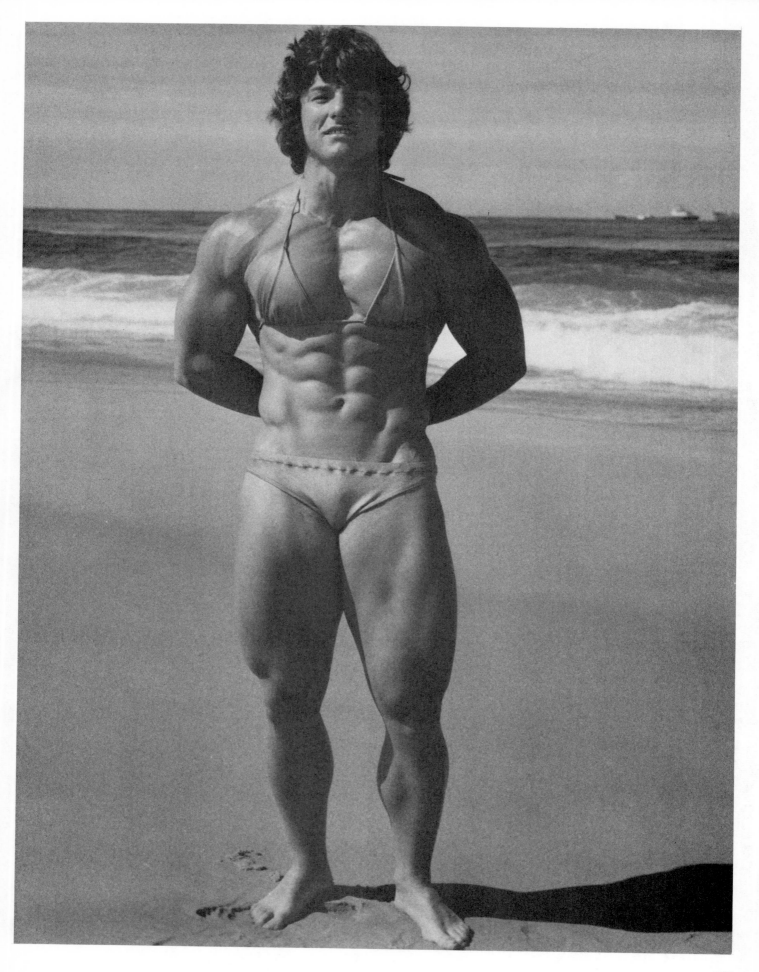

"Bodybuilders should have an aura around them. When you look at a good bodybuilder, you should be awestruck. If you're not awestruck, then the person's body obviously hasn't been developed enough. There hasn't been a perfect woman bodybuilder yet, so you've got to create one in your mind. The body should have a lot of the muscularity of the male bodybuilder, because the muscles on a woman and a man are exactly the same: the same number of muscles, and they're in the same position basically. With a male bodybuilder, there's going to be a bulge in his shorts where the female hasn't got one, and that should be the main distinction. A male bodybuilder should be graceful, should have some elegance in his movement; a woman should also. A male bodybuilder shouldn't be clumsy and awkward; a female bodybuilder shouldn't be clumsy and awkward either. A female bodybuilder will have a female face, which will be a little bit different. My idea of the perfect female bodybuilder is a body that is muscularly as similar to a man as possible, but with the expression and the personality of a female coming out."

—Bev Francis

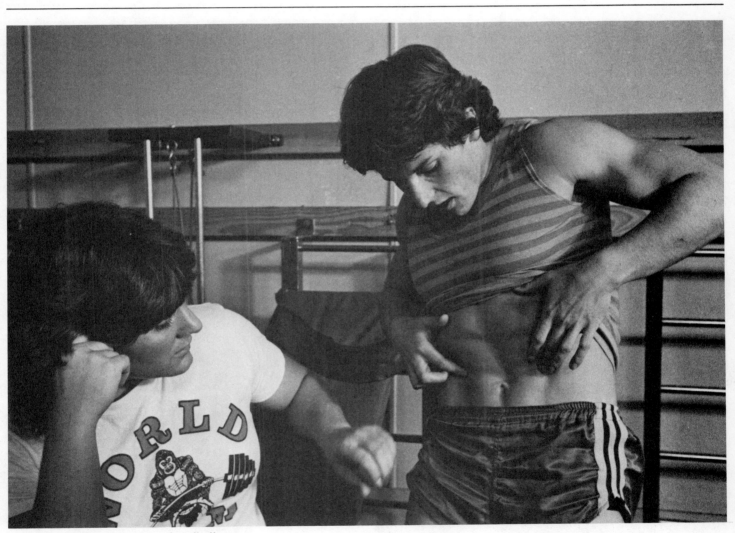

Bev checking her abs with Gail Mulhall

cular woman, and her muscles, in all their visual uncommonness, have come to define her to the outside world.

Now she is on the brink of adopting that definition for herself. While she was a power-lifter, her muscles were a means to an end; for a bodybuilder, they will be an end in themselves, and Bev Francis, in this newest stage of becoming all that she can be, will become what was before a symbol for herself.

A bodybuilder is an identity of sculpted tissue, a self of flesh, and he or she makes a statement of that self on stage in a way that is as profoundly personal as the writing of a poem or the painting of a self-portrait. I wanted before I left Australia to get some idea of what Bev Francis's statement was going to be. I wanted to see her pose, showing her muscles not as power-lifting tools but as the developing components of a new definition of herself, one she would offer, completed, to the world in December at Caesar's Palace. So, shortly after her leg workout in the Football Club Gym, George Butler and I drove her out into the country to a place called Hanging Rock to watch her pose outside, in the harsh light of day.

Hanging Rock is a sort of park, featuring an odd jumble of igneous rock spires rising out of a fragrant koala-bear-populated forest of eucalyptus trees. It was a cool, breezy, cloudy afternoon, but once up among the rocks Bev stripped down to a yellow posing bikini and patiently let George arrange her for photographing at the base of one of the spires. There were a few

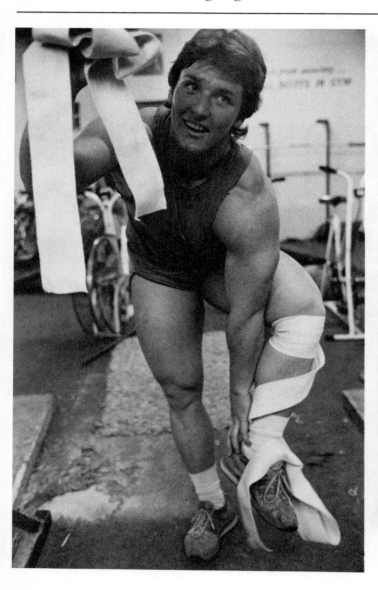

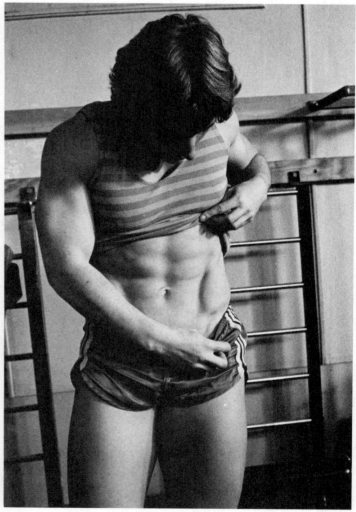

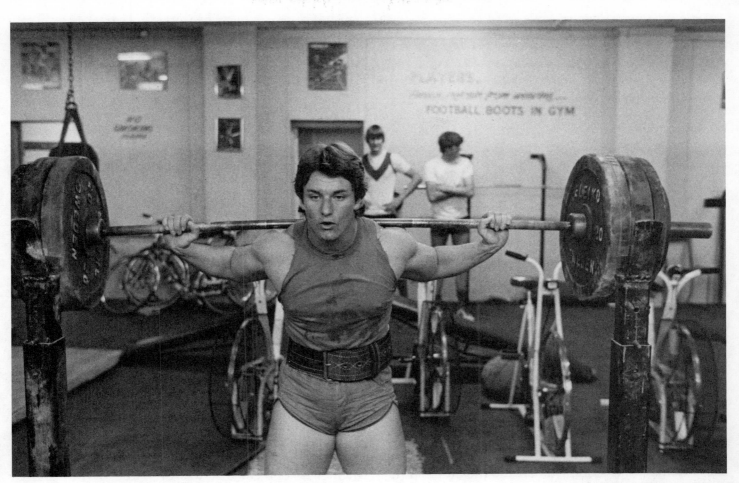

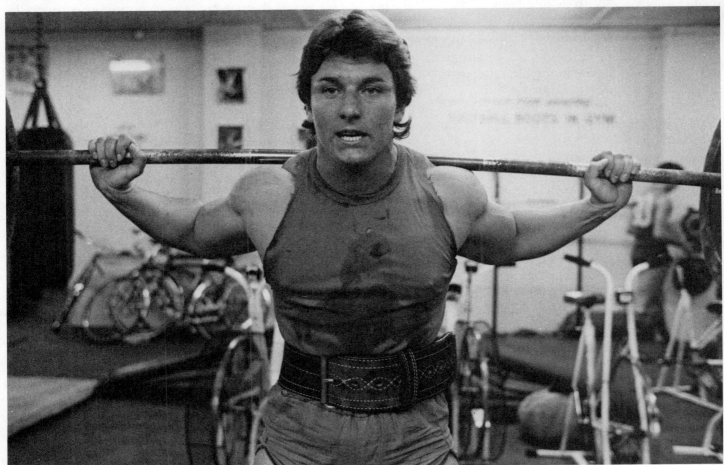

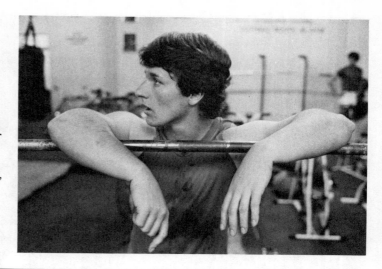

tourists walking around the park taking pictures of rocks, but we drew considerably longer stares from the ones who noticed us. Bev was pale, cold, unoiled and in power-lifting, rather than bodybuilding, shape, but when she began to hit bodybuilding poses in front of the rock spire even one of the koala bears might have known he was seeing something revolutionary.

Whereas the bodies of Cindy Hardee, Rachel McLish, Lynn Conkwright and Kike Elomaa can be seen as interesting—and in some cases beautiful—modifications of the traditional female form, and the bodies of Laura Combes and Carla Dunlap and the other authentically muscular female bodybuilders as somewhat more radically modified versions of that same form, it is all but impossible to see what Bev Francis has made of her physical self as belonging to any female frame of reference at all, traditional or otherwise. When she is posing, her body appears to be not just a quantitative extension of Rachel's or Lynn's, or even of Laura's or Carla's, but something qualitatively different and—because there is no frame of reference for it—existentially unsettling. It is simply not a woman's body, so far as the world and history have prepared us to know what that is. Yet Bev Francis is a woman, not a man, and therefore it is not a man's body either.

She has large, cleanly divided pectoral muscles rather than breasts, and she has no hips. Her arms and shoulders and back are fully, ruggedly developed, and there is not a trace of a traditional female curve in any of those areas. Her stomach is a hard geometry of segmented blocks of abdominal muscles, and the curve of her neck into her shoulders—a curve which almost always remains a concave, "feminine" one on even the most muscular female bodybuilders—is a convex bulge of trapezius muscle.

Her body even now, before being fully defined by bodybuilding training, could place in or win many male bodybuilding contests at state levels or lower—if she were a man. But even in her best bodybuilding shape, I find it hard to believe that Bev will win the 1983 Caesar's Palace competition—because she is a woman, and because women's bodybuilding (like the Englishman on the plane, like most of the rest of the world) is probably not yet prepared to appreciate the statement Bev Francis will make on stage in Las Vegas. It is, as I have said, an unsettling statement, both aesthetically and politically: aesthetically because it refers to no standard other than its own, and politically because it seems to make a particular kind of androgyny the ultimate point of a particular kind of equality between men and women. More important, it is a statement whose main text was prepared by Bev and by Franz Stampfl *outside* of bodybuilding, with no intended reference to the sport to which it has now been adapted. Read into women's bodybuilding from the outside, that uncompromising, unequivocal text becomes revolutionary; and women's bodybuilding, while it will no doubt change aesthetically and politically, will not change overnight by revolution.

But finally, whether she loses or somehow manages to win the contest is less important to the future of women's bodybuilding than her competing in it. (Note: She placed eighth, out of fifteen women.) The sport badly needs ventilation and Beverly May Francis's presence in Las Vegas can't help but open a large window on it. She will be perceived there by some people as a welcome end of the line for the muscular faction of women bodybuilders—a sort of suicidal sine qua non of that aesthetic. But those people will be wrong. Bev Francis is not just Laura Combes carried a little too far, and she is not the end of anything. In fact, George Butler and I both believe that what we found in Melbourne was really just the beginning of a new spectrum—one which very well might contain both the salvation of women's bodybuilding and that elusive American dream known as the New Woman.

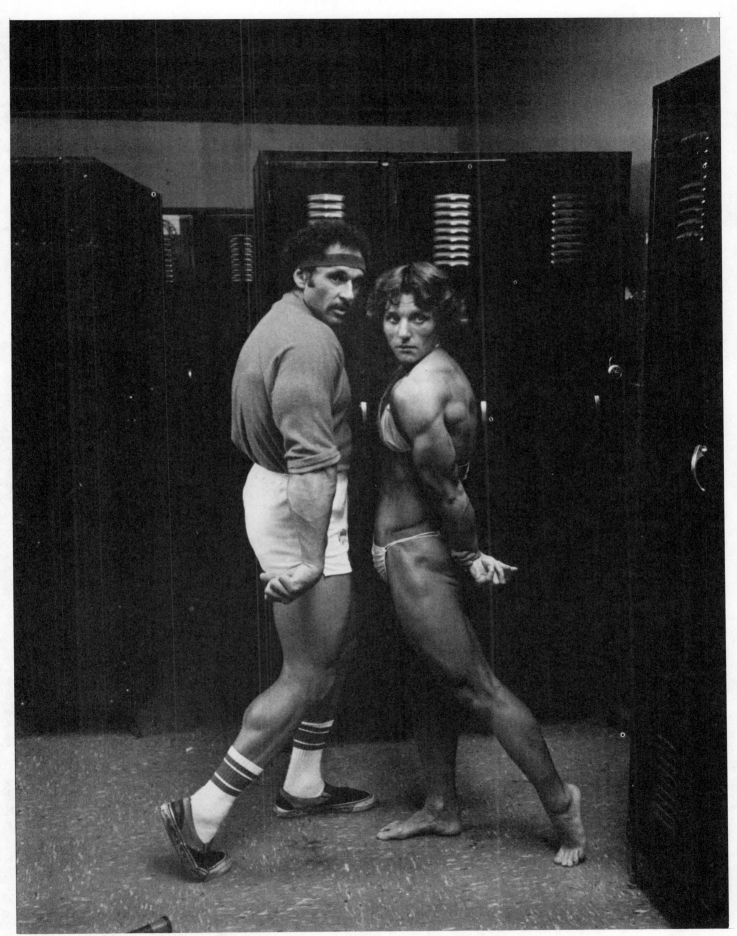

Bev posing with Steve Michalik, preparing for Caesars Cup Competition, Michalik's Gym, 1983

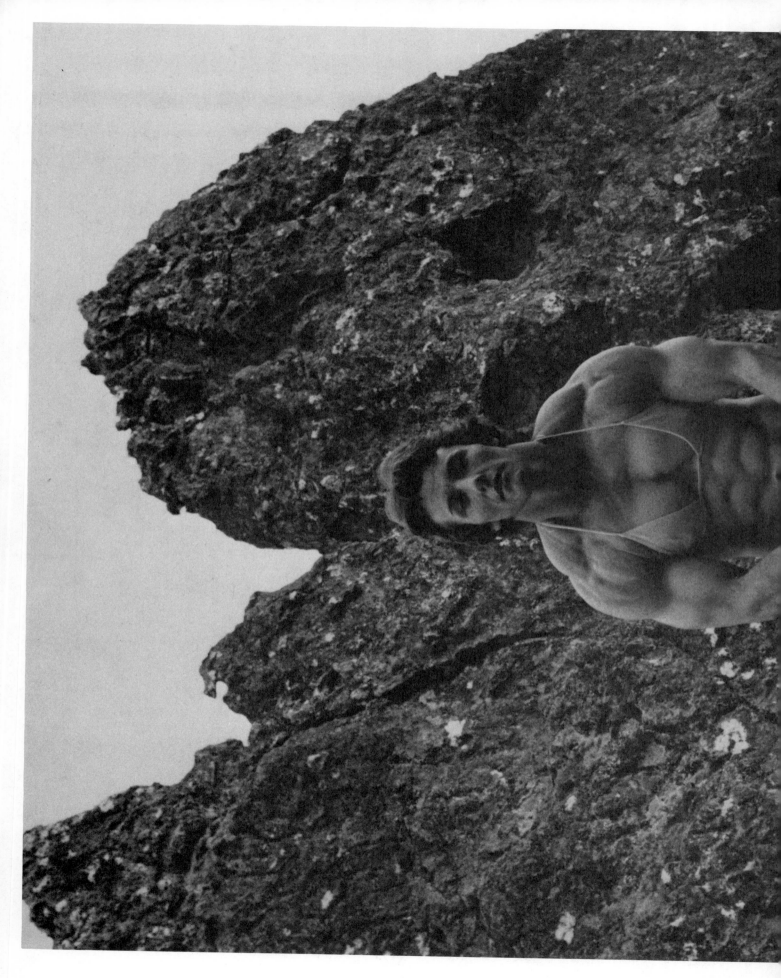

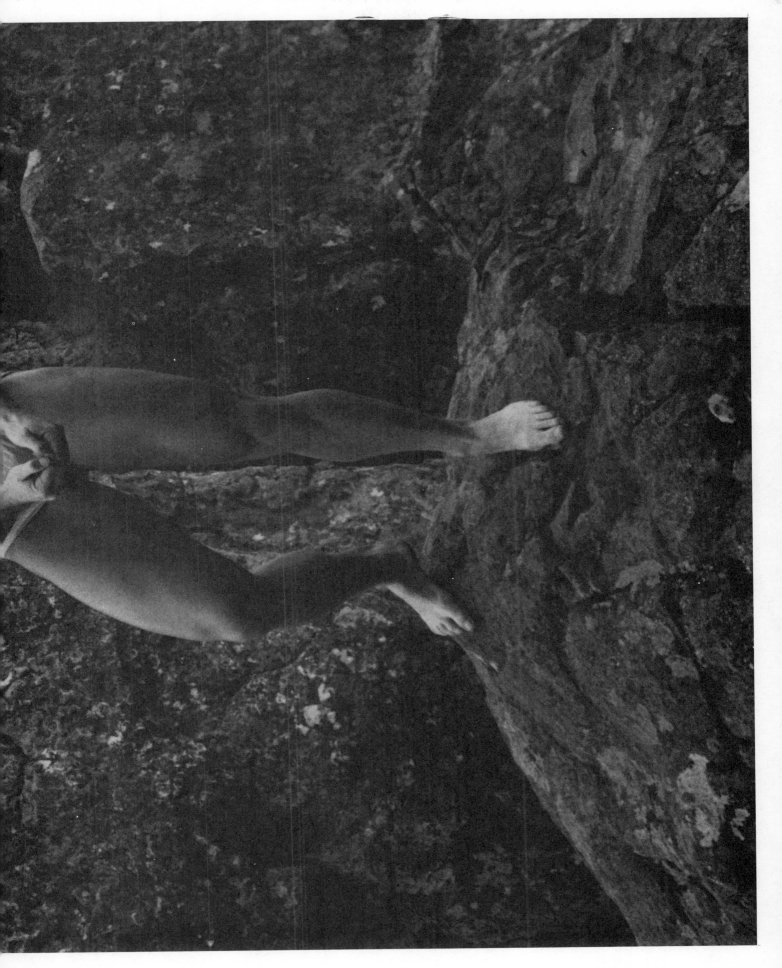

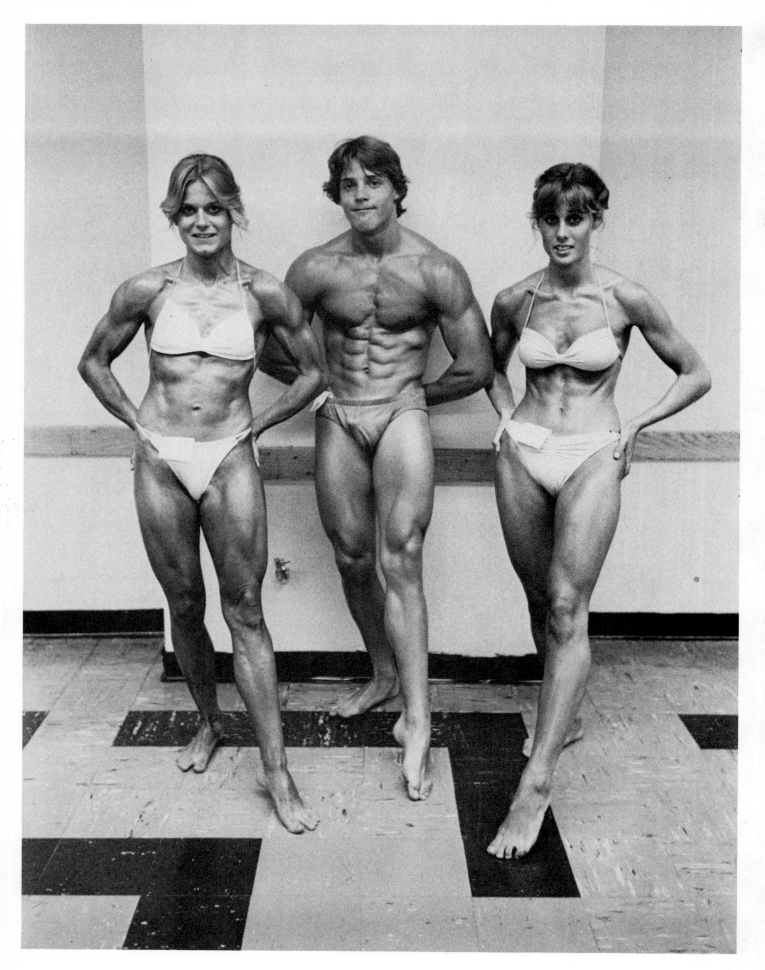

7

It is believed by some that female bodybuilding, still in its infancy, is dying—of a hereditary and untreatable confusion of purposes. Exercise for women, including exercise with weights, has of course never been healthier: there are more women pumping more iron in more gyms now, by far, than at any time in history. But competitive women's bodybuilding, the contesting onstage of female musculature, is, according to some, already moribund after only two years of real life.

How could that be so?

For a spectator sport to thrive in this country, there has to be money in it. Until recently there was no money to speak of in male bodybuilding and that sport languished until the emergence of Arnold Schwarzenegger, the book and film versions of *Pumping Iron,* and the national health and beauty boom, all of the past ten years, pulled it back to life. There is money in male bodybuilding now because, for whatever reasons, Americans currently approve of muscles on men and are willing to pay to see them—because, to put it even more simply, enough men want to look like bodybuilders and because enough women find them sexy.

It is widely believed among the powers that be in female bodybuilding that *real* muscles on women, the unequivocal, bulging, Bev Francis kind of muscles ordinarily associated with men, are not salable in America—that the great majority of women do not want them and that the great majority of men are threatened or appalled or disgusted by them, and that even though people may pay once or twice out of curiosity to see those kinds of muscles on women, they will not continue to pay to see them. The powers that be may be right about that, and they may not be. It is possible that we will never know for sure, because in the sport's effort to make itself commercially viable, women's bodybuilding tends more and more to hide the women who own that kind of muscles, the Laura Combeses and Lisa Elliotts and Mary Robertses and Auby Paulicks and Cammie Luskos and Debbie Basiles.

For whatever reasons, those women do not win the major contests, do not endorse the major bodybuilding products, do not sit on the committees and federations which control female bodybuilding, and are less and less featured in the magazines which report and advertise the sport. They are kept on the sidelines, those women with big muscles, and women's bodybuilding is now almost totally represented and embodied by slim, athletic, graceful, pretty women—the Rachels and Lynns and Candys and Kikes—on whom muscles do not show until they are flexed and then only demurely, and with whom, it is hoped by those with a commercial interest in the sport, American women will want to identify and American men will want to dally.

Ironically, it is precisely this survival strategy being employed by women's bodybuilding which the doomsayers believe is killing it. The sport, they say, has returned to the old days of the Miss Americana contests with skinnier contestants, and consists now of a series of vapid beauty contests among women with the taut, fatless, slightly desiccated bodies of female gymnasts, which no one in his or her right mind would pay to go to more than once. How, these doomsayers ask, can you all but require, for aesthetic or commercial or whatever reasons, that competitors in the sport go only so far, develop themselves only up to a point and not beyond it, and still expect their competitions to interest anyone? By analogy, how much interest would there be in a series of hundred-yard dashes in which all the runners had agreed (or been persuaded) never to finish in under ten seconds?

Those are good, relevant questions, and it is likely that if female bodybuilding is to flourish it will have to address them and, through them, the deeper question of what the sport and art of women's bodybuilding are all about. Are they all about the showing off onstage of healthy, fit, marketable women to no particular end other than that? Or are they about the unhindered development and competition of female muscle?

Though a majority of the present legislators and promoters of women's bodybuilding appear to find that second option unsettling, not to mention financially impractical, they very well may be soon stuck with having to make the best of it. And that could be the making of the sport—for in that second definitive possibility, quite aside from its marketing problems, there is the mysterious potential for growth, both physical and symbolic; there is resonance that is at the same time political, sociological and historic; and there is an opportunity, perhaps the only one, for women's bodybuilding to finally find its archetype.

No one wishes all those things more fervently for women's bodybuilding than Al Thomas, a fifty-two-year-old English professor at a Pennsylvania college, who is to women's bodybuilding and weight training more or less what Homer was to war. Since 1961 he has written over a hundred articles on the subject for *Iron Man, Muscular Development, Body and Power* and other bodybuilding magazines. Despite a certain talent for writing and a total command of the subject, he has not tried to publish his articles in more general interest magazines because, he says, he writes to influence people *within* the sport, not outside it.

Al Thomas is interested in influence because he is a man with a theme; his theme is, and has been for twenty years, the glory of muscular womanhood. Though he can and does write lyrically and at length about the purely physical beauty of women with mus-

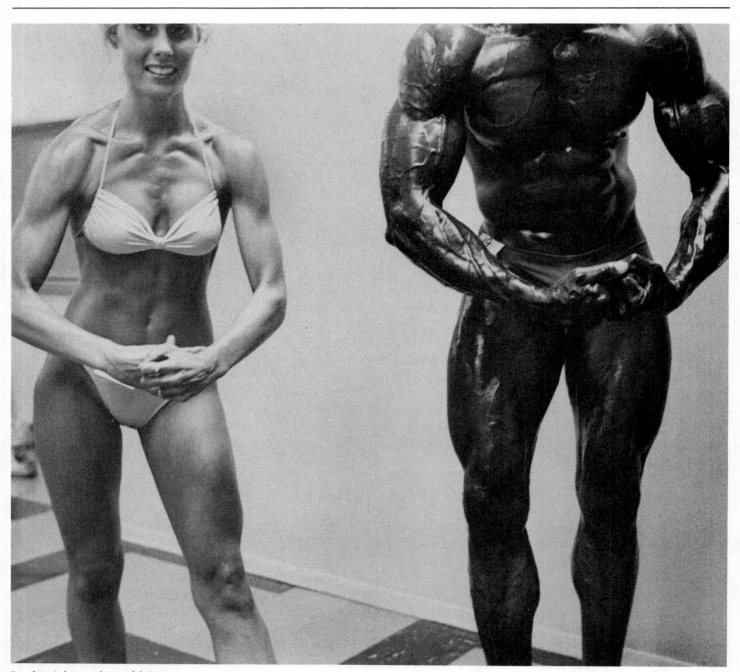

Cynthia Sabia and Arnold Caesar

cles, Thomas saves his most passionate writing for the political and cultural implications of female muscles, and the absence of them. He loathes what he calls the "Hollywood glamour queen" body—the Betty Grable, Miss America, thin-shanked, soft-armed, slack-bellied look, a look he refers to frequently as clinically atrophied—not only because he finds it unexciting visually but also for what it has to say about the condition of women: "Beauty queen shows give expression to what a middle-class society and a coterie of tired old men think is 'appropriate,' 'cute,' and above all unthreatening.

"Muscles have been admired in all of God's creatures but one: the human female," says Al Thomas. And in the fact that they have not been admired in her, he

"In a posing routine you have to have different emotions, like you want to be muscular, you want some poses to be sexy and alluring with the chest back. You have to add a little in your posing routine, but that is planned and it's there for a purpose. But then I step right out and do a really hard core muscle shot followed by a semi-cheesecake, sexy shot. I do include a couple of these poses in it that aren't too obvious—just a slight hint. But as far as on stage, like the poseoff, it's muscularity I just try to show my physique to the best."
—Rachel McLish

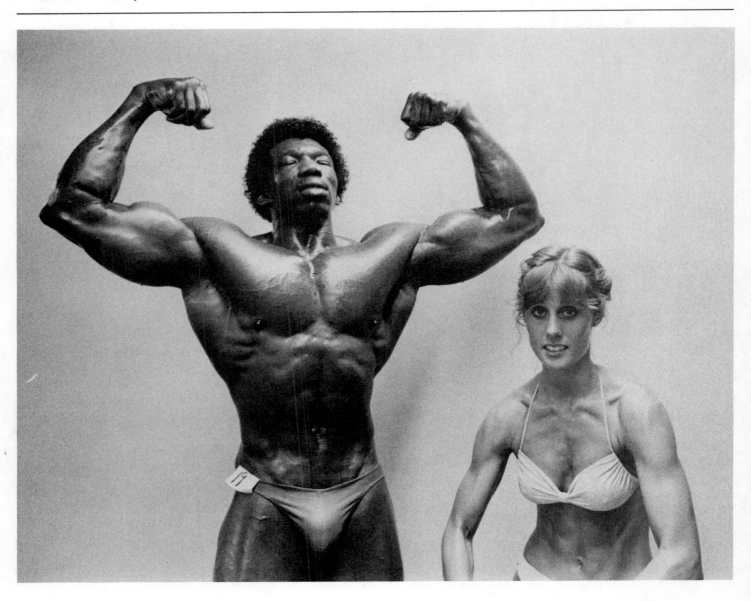

finds a world of male repression and fear. "The symbolizing faculty being what it is," he wrote in an article entitled "Some Notes toward an Aesthetics of Body for the Modern Woman," "woman's body and flesh and muscle have always been feared as objective correlatives for a sexual potential vaguely apprehended by the adult male—and presaged by the boy—as an implicit threat to him as an individual, rather than as a member of a sex. . . . Hence the need to divest woman of her flesh."

Women's bodybuilding, Thomas believes, is, on its most significant level, a means of reclaiming that flesh and, at the same time, of staking out a new and ultimate kind of freedom for it. He not only believes this, he believes it *passionately* and vividly—his head evi-

"So that's always been a real thing with me, you know, to prove to people that you can actually have a muscular physique but be feminine."
—Lynn Conkwright

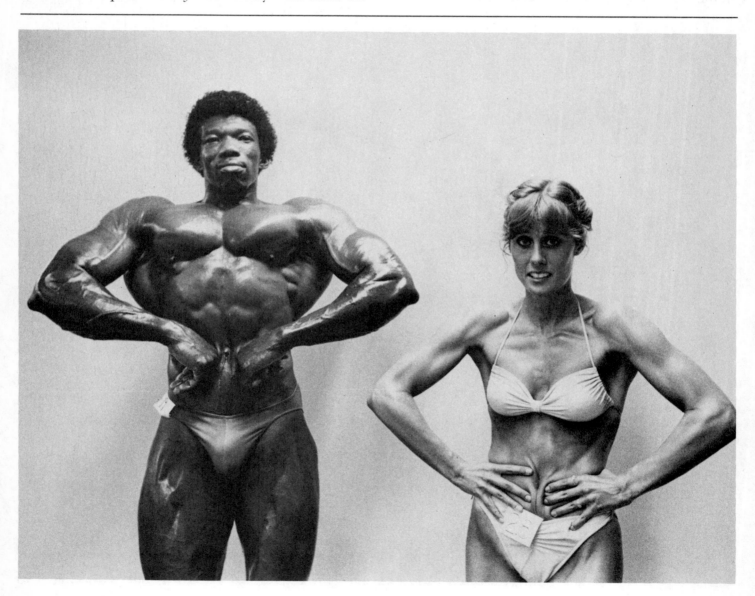

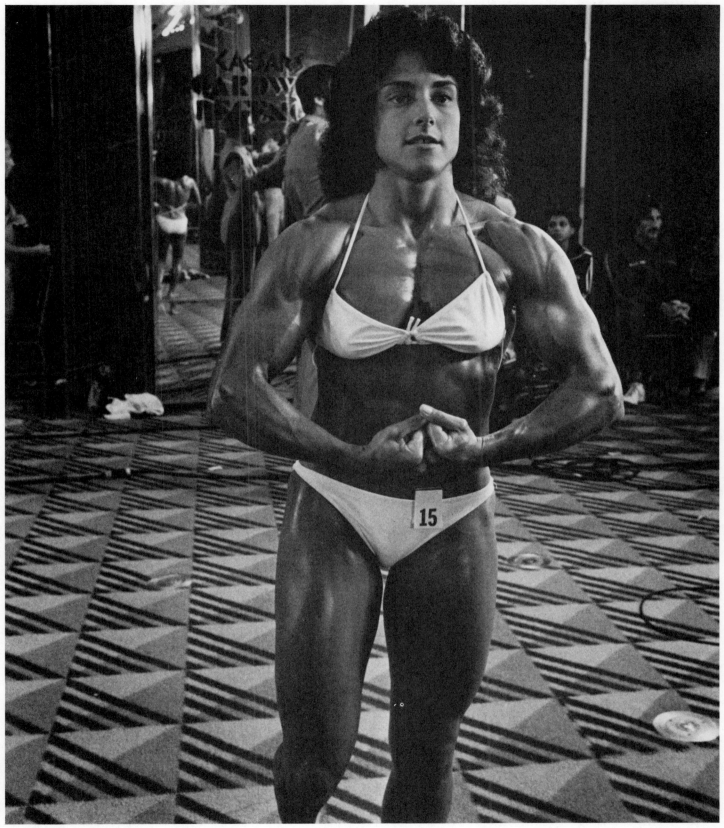

Laura Combes

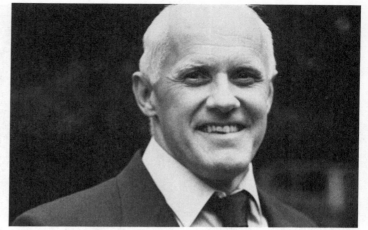
Al Thomas

dently full of the actual lineaments of that free and reclaimed flesh—and if his writing on the subject is occasionally a little stiff and obscure, that passion is always near the surface, ready to break through dissonantly and interestingly, as it does here:

The real signs of woman's exploitation are not inequitable abortion laws and policies of matriculation or hiring. Even the painfully frustrating sexual role to which she has been conditioned by centuries of manipulation by shaman and priest (inglorious decline from the reign of *magna mater,* big breasted and stout of thigh), even this is merely symptomatic of a larger disorder. Woman's malaise, the anger which has sparked the present revolution, grows out of her unawareness not only about what her body is, but about what body is. . . . For woman to "know" herself, to discern with the living flesh of her hand the mysteries of the living flesh that is she, she must be a breaker of the little Gods of the hearthside who have exacted her womanliness as the price of their propitiation. Her meatness is she, and there is no definition of her— however high flown its accounting of soul, *anima,* breath, spirit—that can properly fail to grapple with the aesthetic-religious problem that consciousness terminates in flesh. . . . Woman strong in the flesh has wakened *to* body, not *from* body. Fulfillment, in both the religious and aesthetic senses, is not an idea, but incarnate thingness, in body. . . .

Incarnate woman, not disjunct, not fragmented, solid square-hipped meat bearer. With hardly a place to lay her head, with hardly a free man to seed her womb. But free.

It is difficult but tempting to imagine women reading this in little gyms all over the world, women like Bev Francis who are not yet world-class bodybuilders but who see in Al Thomas's abstruse, excited prose a method and reason for getting there. For the fact is that Al Thomas is and has been telling women's bodybuilding (or that part of it which can read him and is not already too angered by him to do so) what is best and most interesting about itself. And most revolutionary, for if Thomas is the sport's Homer he is also its Mao and its Che. "Clench your fists when you pose,

dammit," he is telling those yet undiscovered stout-thighed women in little gyms. "Be proud of your muscle, your incarnate freedom, by God. Don't hold back, no matter what the establishment tells you. It's too important! Go for everything you can!"

Listen to Al Thomas once again, waxing passionate this time on the subject of women's arms and their symbolism, and on the revolutionary theme of growth through resistance:

Shape (form) is the arms' response to resistance. In human beings (as opposed to Hollywood "glamour queens") this shape (form) is predictable, including for the female no less than the male a range of delicious hillocks referred to as deltoids, triceps, biceps, and brachialis—all tapering off into that crisscrossing network of gulleys and ravines known as the forearm. . . .

Less figuratively, most movie queens' arms simply bear no resemblance to natural constructs. In nature, things are wild and untamed; they run riot. Even untrained natural arms are a riot of sinews, vein systems, and muscle configurations. In short, they are alive. Things come to life beneath the flesh when the arm is lifted, when it embraces, when it implores. For all her imploring, the movie queen's arm is silent, expressing nothing, giving no sense of things alive and working beneath the flesh. Indeed it is the viewer's awareness of the indulgent flesh's not being commanded or shaped by sinew and muscle that leaves him or her with a sense of "moral sag" and insipidity, rather than just the sense of fleshly sag and the drooping away from the bone of sick flesh. . . .

The arm as vine is the inevitable contrivance of a society which see females as creatures whose function is to cling. To those with a larger view of woman, such a view of any human being is demeaning. Womanly muscularity is a badge of vigor in a society that still too often prefers its women of a doughier consistency, both morally and physically.

If that isn't an eloquent call to arms, I'd like to know what is.

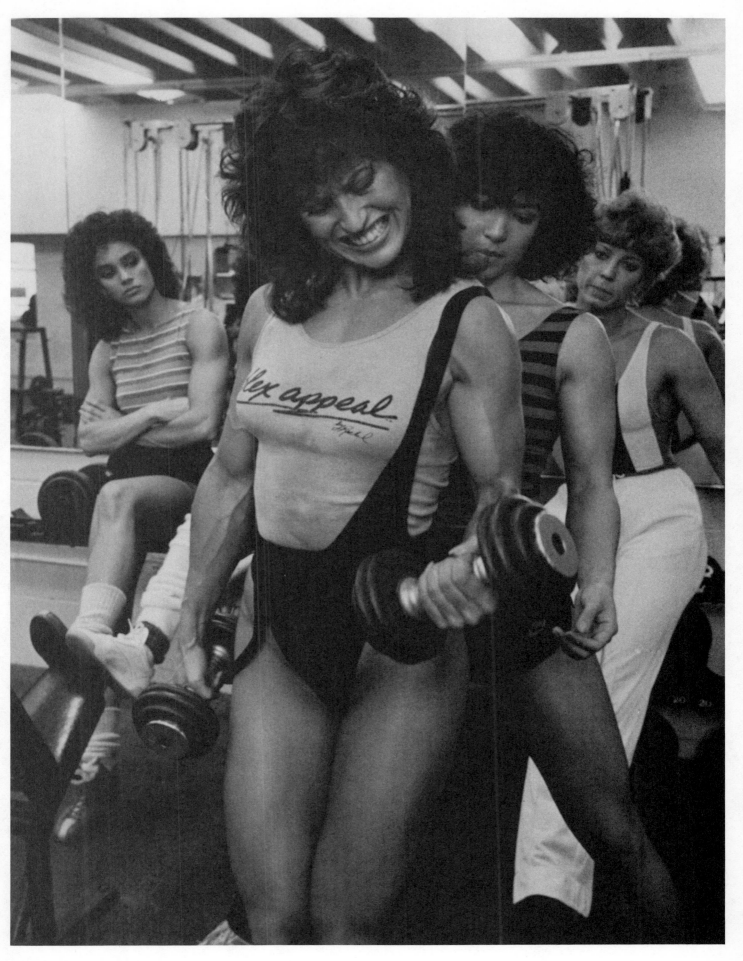

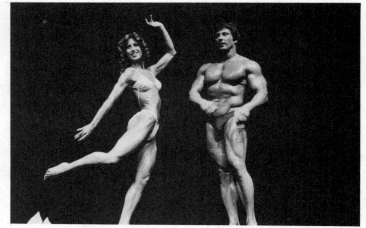

Rachel with Frank Zane

Al Thomas says she must be a "large woman, in spirit as well as body. Our heroes are always large. She would show what it is really like to be a woman—courageous, generous, free in spirit, unafraid. She would be an embodiment of all the metaphors of female strength."

He is talking here about Superwoman, the as yet undiscovered, or unmade, ultimate woman bodybuilder. Thomas believes in her and so do I. In my mind too she is large. She is five feet ten and weighs one hundred and fifty pounds, and there is nothing at all demure about her physique. She has perfect proportions and such overall symmetry that your eye is never distracted by a particular part but sees each movement she makes as an expression of the whole, and rests centered on her when she is still, as the eye does on the symmetry of an egg or a Doric column. Within her symmetry each muscle group, calves and thighs, waist and back, chest, shoulders and arms, is developed to its maximum potential, beyond any development we have ever seen on a woman. The muscles show themselves in repose and are as natural-looking on her, whether flexed or unflexed, as the muscles of a thoroughbred mare or a female lion. Fully developed as these muscles are, they do not look masculine. In their naturalness and perfect proportion to one another, they look neither masculine nor feminine, only exactly correct on her, correct to the point of necessity: even though nothing like it has been seen before, it is impossible to imagine her physique composed in any other way. That physique has this, and maybe only this, in common with those of most current women bodybuilders: it is not sexually stimulating. Created with no reference to male fantasies, it does not invite them. But it does move everyone who sees it; like all unique art, it seems to surprise and gratify at the same time, and to commence, instantaneously, its own history.

It is in this imagined woman, and only in her, that both the reality and the promise of women's body-building can meet, and in whom its future can be guaranteed. She is coming. If she is not here already, undiscovered, she soon will be. And she will be something to see. In the manner in which she has created herself, without reference to men and their fantasies, she will be claiming a sort of freedom and self-realization unique to women since prehistoric matriarchal societies. In that way she will be an extension of current women bodybuilders, who to the degree that they are now shaping themselves unhindered by biological obligation, historical precedent, and tastes other than their own, are already doing something culturally unique. She will be an extension too of the woman-as-doer in America, of every Amelia Earhart and Babe Zaharias and Jane Fonda, every female Little Leaguer and truck driver and trauma surgeon and judge in our society who has bashed her way through sexual stereotyping and gone on to do what she wanted to do. But this woman will also be something unextended and brand new under the sun: a new archetype; a woman so uniquely and totally self-made that in all of history there is no design for her.

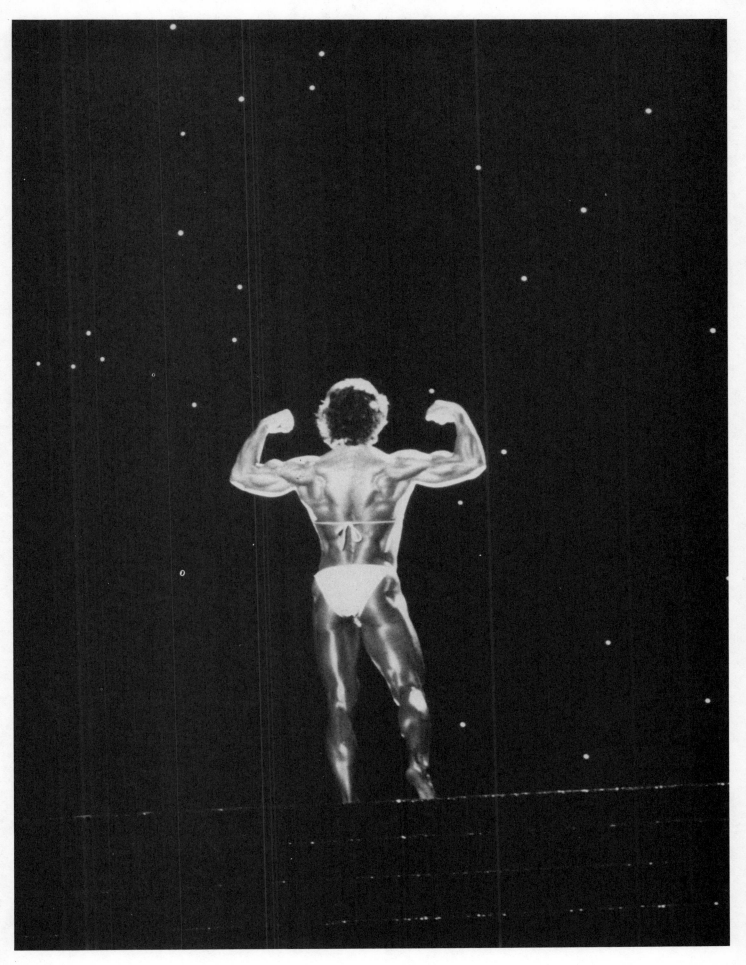

George Butler is a photographer and filmmaker who lives on a farm in the White Mountains of New Hampshire. He was co-editor of *The New Soldier* and the producer/director who made the movies *Pumping Iron* and *Pumping Iron II—The Women*.

Charles Gaines lives with his wife, Patricia, and three children on top of a ledge in New Hampshire. He leaves there as infrequently as possible.

All photographs in this book (with the exception of the historical material) were taken with a Leica M4 camera and a leitz summilux 1.4 35MM lense. Throughout I use Kodak Tri-X film with available light only.

All historical photos from the collection of Orrin Heller–Box 301, Norwalk, CA 90650